Who Said I'd Never Dance Again?

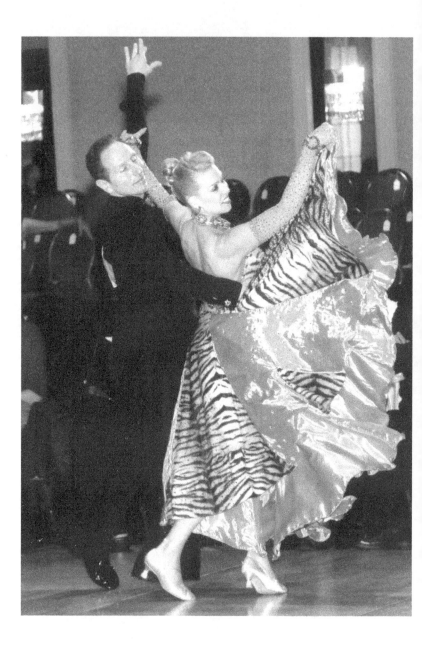

# Who Said I'd Never Dance Again?

## A Journey From Hip Replacement Surgery To Athletic Victory

# Darla Davies

Including inspirational stories of perseverance and comeback

**Foreword by World's Leading Sports Psychologist Dr. Bob Rotella**

NEW YORK

LONDON • NASHVILLE • MELBOURNE • VANCOUVER

# Who Said I'd Never Dance Again?

## A Journey from Hip Replacement Surgery to Athletic Victory

Published in New York, New York, by Morgan James Publishing. Morgan James is a trademark of Morgan James, LLC. www.MorganJamesPublishing.com

ISBN 9781642790917 paperback
ISBN 9781642790924 eBook
Library of Congress Control Number: 2018945739

**Cover and Interior Design by:**
Chris Treccani
www.3dogcreative.net

**Editing and author support:**
Tanya Brockett, Hallagen Ink

**Photos:**
Park West Photography, Ryan Kenner Photography,
Dore Studios, and Deca Dance Photography

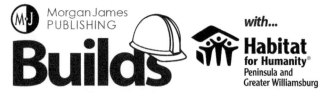

Morgan James is a proud partner of Habitat for Humanity Peninsula and Greater Williamsburg. Partners in building since 2006.

Get involved today! Visit
MorganJamesPublishing.com/giving-back

To my husband, Jim: My mentor, my teacher, my best friend, and my love. Thank you for your steadfast belief, support, and encouragement through my surgery, recovery, and return to dancing.

To my surgeon, Dr. Anthony Hedley, who from day one was honest, to the point, positive, and encouraging. Your warm smile and confidence gave me comfort and hope.

# *Contents*

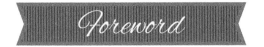
# Foreword

"Believe you can win."
**—Dr. Bob Rotella**

For an athlete to succeed in whatever sport they play, they have to allow their mind to lead their body to do what it knows to do to be successful. When they can learn to love their sport, accept the good with the bad, and become what I call "unconscious" when they play, they will excel. Being unconscious is getting your conscious mind out of the way (the mechanics or technical game) so your mental and physical routine has the opportunity to pay off in your actions. You let go and enjoy what it is you are doing and your body does what it knows to do.

Getting the mental game in line can be a bigger challenge for athletes who have faced physical challenges like major surgery or joint replacement. Not only does the athlete have to deal with the physical discomfort of the ailment that lead to surgery and subsequent recovery, but they have to overcome the negative mental impact that surgery has had on their mental game. That doubt and fear can creep into their minds and tell them that they are washed up and won't be able to take that title again. As I have said in my presentations, it doesn't matter if it's the best players in the world or you, you don't have a chance when you let fear or doubt control or rule you. Since your mind tends to control your body, you have to take on the right mental attitude about your ability to let your talent shine, regardless of the setbacks you have to overcome.

In this book, Darla Davies shares how the physical and emotional pain of hip replacement surgery has the potential to create huge obstacles to post-operative success for an athlete. Where many athletes have had to give up their dreams of championship play after joint replacement, Darla chose to buy into what her mind said about her chances of success, and her body fell in line with that belief. Success is an attitude, and athletes facing hip replacement surgery need to keep their attitudes positive and believe in their own talents if they want to succeed. This is the defining moment, where one's mental attitude either drives the desire to pursue the dream, or causes one to walk away and give up on the dream.

As a sidelined athlete, Darla showed the passion for her sport of dancing, along with the desire to come back and set new goals. She showed determination in her fight to regain fitness through rehabilitation therapy and strength training. Darla dared to believe in her dream of winning again after hip replacement with her positive, enthusiastic attitude, and perseverance.

Darla's story of determination and resiliency will inspire and give hope to anyone who might be facing joint-replacement surgery. Darla's quest for athletic victory will show all athletes that it is never too late, and you are never too old to pursue your dream.

**—Dr. Bob Rotella**
Sports psychologist and best-selling author
www.drbobrotella.com

# Preface

"You have to believe there's something at the other side. And you have to have faith in yourself. You have to think that you have the tools to accomplish it."

**—Twyla Tharp**

The purpose of this book is to alleviate the apprehensions and fears in those of you who are facing hip replacement surgery. Perhaps you are someone who has suffered through months or even years of hip pain. Perhaps you have been misled or uninformed as to what is actually causing your back or leg pain. My intention is for my story to help you to avoid the rocky road of pain, misinformation, false hope, and depression caused by a deteriorating hip joint. You will see that there is hope for eliminating your joint pain, and quite possibly, an even better life for you on the other side of surgery.

By the year 2030, hip replacements will increase from over 280,000 now, to over 570,000. You might be surprised to find out that many of your friends and acquaintances have had joint replacement surgery. For many, an active lifestyle does not have to end after a hip replacement. Artificial hip joints have been so successful that people are able to return to the golf course, tennis courts, and dance floor only a few months after surgery. This surgery can actually give one back an active, joyful life at any age, and in many cases, a far better quality of life than what one had experienced prior to surgery. It is possible for hip replacement recipients to emerge from this experience stronger than ever, with a confidence, and a belief that new achievements are possible. Even if you are over fifty, with an artificial hip, athletic victory does not have to be merely a dream; it can be a real possibility.

In addition to chronicling my own journey through hip replacement surgery and recovery, I will share with you the inspiring and amazing recovery and comeback stories of several well-known athletes and dancers. Instead of accepting the end of a celebrated career, these individuals demonstrated the drive and fight to make impressive and unprecedented reemergence into their professional arenas.

In addition to explaining the physical disadvantages and the emotional feelings of trying to return to sport competition with an artificial hip, I will delve into the psychological pressures on competitive dancers and athletes. What roadblocks do they encounter in the pursuit of victory? What does it take to win a United States championship title in the sport of ballroom dancing? Can an athlete with an artificial hip win such a title? You will find the answers to these questions on the pages that follow.

# Acknowledgments

Tanya Brockett, Editor & Publishing Mentor—Much gratitude for your encouragement and support throughout this journey. I appreciate your expertise, your commitment, and your persistence. You always believed in me and knew that this book would one day inspire many others to persevere through their challenges. Thank you.

Morgan James Publishing—What a gift to have been introduced to and to work with a highly competent and equally lovely group of individuals. A special thank you to David Hancock (Morgan James CEO and founder), Jim Howard, Aubrey Kosa, Bonnie Rauch, and Terry Whalin for your professionalism and support through the process.

## Chapter 1

# Renewed Passion and Intense Pain

People tend to look at dancers like we are these little jewels, little cardboard cutouts, and yet we have blood and guts and go through hell.

**—Susan Jaffe**

My osteoarthritis had probably been creeping up on me for a few years. Unaware of the origin and cause of the ache in my groin area, I assumed that it was just the muscle strain experienced by any athlete. I thought that if I soaked my legs in a bath of Epsom salts, and used topical pain-relieving creams, I could manage and control my pain.

I had participated in so many sports activities over the years that occasional leg and back pain was expected as part of the program. I had spent countless hours in the saddle going over jumps during more than twenty-five years of equestrian competitions. In addition, I had spent many years trying to improve my golf and tennis skills. I grimace now as I recall all of that sprinting and quick shuffling back and forth on the tennis court. All of that stop and start action probably had a huge impact on my disappearing joint cartilage. Years of daily gym workouts reflected my commitment to improving my strength and stamina for my various sporting endeavors.

Horses had always been my first love, but after years of experiencing the thrill of equestrian competition, along with the efforts and expenses of the business, I finally got burned out on the whole "horsey" thing.

When I had been totally enmeshed in my horse-crazy life, I had zero interest in even watching ballroom dancing when it was on television. Finding myself horseless for the first time in twenty-five years, I felt like a huge chunk of my life was missing, and I was yearning for a new passion. I really liked both tennis and golf, but neither sport took the place in my heart that the horses had dominated for all of those years in my past.

I finally got around to watching a few of those televised dance competitions. They ignited a spark of intrigue and interest in me. This was obviously more than just regular dancing: the fit bodies, the costumes, the speed, the strength, the skill, and the showmanship. Wow! One competition that I watched on ESPN was even called the "DanceSport Championships." *No kidding!* I thought. This kind of dancing was every bit of a sport and more! Feeling completely mesmerized by the highly skilled, dancing athletes, and all of the glitz, I wondered, *could I do that?*

I started taking swing dance lessons at a community center, and eventually found a small ballroom dance studio where I realized my new passion. I wanted to become a competitive amateur ballroom dancer. I learned that ballroom dance competitions offered many levels of participation, from newcomer through advanced, as well as numerous age divisions.

After a couple years of learning in small local dance studios, fate led me to meet my husband-to-be, Jim Maranto, former two-time United States Professional American Smooth Ballroom Dance Champion.

That is when my real dance education began. I became a good student; one who was always anxious to learn and excel at the competitions. I progressed from beginner through intermediate to the advanced level of competition within a period of about five years.

Most people do not realize the amount of leg strength and foot articulation required for high-level ballroom dancing—a dancer uses the standing leg to transfer body weight to the other leg. The Rhythm and Latin styles of dancing require movement of the rib cage, as well as hip rotation, which produces that exciting Cuban hip action. Good dancers have a "grounded" quality, showing strong foot pressure against the floor as they move.

I found that I was using my legs and my body more in ballroom dancing than I ever had in any other sport. It seemed as though my legs and my feet were perpetually sore. Over the years my left leg pain grew to be more severe; it traveled from the groin area, down behind my knee, and even down the front of my lower leg. If I picked up my right foot, standing with all of my weight on my left leg, I could hear my left knee making cracking noises.

My dancing skills were improving and I was doing very well at competitions. However, my joint pain was growing more intense as time marched on. In spite of the fact that I did not have tremendous leg strength, I was successful because other elements of my overall dance performance and presentation either made up for or disguised this weakness. I feared that at some point my secret vulnerability would become obvious to the critical eyes of the competition judging panels. I was concerned, but did not know how worried I should be. Was this leg pain serious? Was I doomed? Or was it fixable?

Several of my dancing buddies had raved to me about this Rolfer who had worked wonders on their body pains. I knew of dancers who used massage therapists regularly, but I had never heard of Rolfing. I was told Rolfing was like a deep tissue massage. Willing to try anything, I signed up for a session with "Bill the Rolfer," as he was known at our dance studio. Bill explained to me that Rolfing works on the connective tissues (facia) that surround, support, and penetrate our muscles, bones, nerves, and organs. The goal of Rolfing is to release, realign, and balance the whole body, thus improving posture and freedom of movement. Ultimately, Rolfing can potentially eliminate discomfort by alleviating tension and pain.

Let me just say that Rolfing is not for sissies! I was determined to hang in there for several sessions. I told Bill that I feared there might be hip replacement surgery in my future. Bill was optimistic that my pain, along with the need for surgery, would be gone after he got my leg bones un-jammed and more aligned. After a few Rolfing sessions, I did see some improvement in my body alignment, posture, balance, and flexibility, but my nagging groin pain continued.

*Oh, where to now? Which way should I go?* I thought. I recalled Dorothy in the *Wizard of Oz*, when she came to a fork in the yellow brick road. She looked up at the scarecrow, and he told her she could either go "this way," "that way," or "both ways." I was feeling frustrated and lost. I had to find someone who could get rid of my pain. I needed to find a wizard.

I decided to make an appointment with a chiropractor my friends recommended. The chiropractor assured me that the groin pain I described was not caused by a hip problem. Looking at my X-ray, he confirmed that I had something unusual, found in one out of every five thousand people. It is called "sacralization," which occurs when the two bottom lumbar vertebra on each side of the spine are actually fused to the pelvic bone. This triangular bone at the bottom of the spine, called the sacrum, is connected to the two hipbones through the sacroiliac joints. One positive for me was that both of the vertebras on each side of my spine were fused to the pelvic bone, instead of just being connected on one side or the other.

The chiropractor also pointed out that my spine is somewhat curved and my pelvis is crooked. *Yikes!* I thought. I wondered how these conditions had not caused me any pain when participating in various sports over the past forty-five years. From ballet to flipping on trampolines and off of diving boards to swinging around uneven parallel bars to riding horses for all of those years to leaping through the air at tennis balls to swinging a golf club, I had never felt any restriction of movement due to this so called sacralization. How, after all those years of activity, could these conditions now be causing my intense groin ache?

Even when I mentioned to the chiropractor that my mother had had a hip replacement, he still maintained that my pain was not due to hip problems, and he assured me that chiropractic care would help to alleviate my pain. Looking back, I have to wonder why a specific hip X-ray was not done or even suggested. I guess that I had just assumed that the chiropractor had examined my hip joints on the X-ray, as well as my spine and pelvic bones. Much later, I would learn that my assumption was incorrect.

I wanted so much to believe that this chiropractic treatment could be a quick-fix solution to my problem. I needed something to believe in, because I was not going to let anything stop me from competing in the upcoming United States DanceSport Championships. My left leg had to hold up for another five months. Having placed second in this event the previous year, I was lusting for victory and determined to compete at these national championships.

Over those next five months, I had many chiropractic treatments. Although I had a great attitude and wanted to believe that I was improving, my pain was still present and only worsening.

One day I was walking in the mall and suddenly my leg just felt like it got locked up or jammed in my groin area. It was frightening because the pain was so severe. I was not sure I was going to be able to walk all the way back to my car. I guess I sort of walked my way through that episode that day, but that same painful, locked-up groin feeling would continue to present itself now and then. Not often enough, however, to make me quit dancing.

I continued to believe that I was going to find some doctor who would solve my pain problem. Merely walking and getting myself in and out of the car was painful. I was unable to dance in practice or competition without over-the-counter pain medication. In addition to the groin pain, my knee began to feel weak and painful as well. I was falling apart, and I knew it, but I was still not ready to throw in the towel. I started wearing a knee brace for both dance practices and competitions. I knew that masking the pain was not a solution, but heck, it was working, and the pills and supportive bandages were serving a purpose to keep me going until I could find the wizard who would be my savior.

I did not know much about acupuncture, but had read positive reports in a few health magazines. The only firsthand knowledge I had about the treatment was when one of my dad's racehorses had been treated with acupuncture. After the treatment where these long needles had been stuck into the horse's back, his racing performance actually did improve. The idea did seem a bit far-fetched to me, but I felt like I had to give acupuncture a chance so I could say that I had left no stone unturned. Like everything else, I wanted to believe that the acupuncture was going to be my magic cure; however, it turned out to be nothing more beneficial than a few hours of nice music and relaxation.

In spite of my joint and leg pain, I was able to press on with the dancing for the next few months. I kept my legs limber by riding the recumbent stationary bike for thirty minutes every day, and my over-the-counter "friends" helped me get through short dance practices. Every night, I put ice packs on my hip and my knee, and then I sat with my lower legs in my electric foot massager for thirty minutes. I refused to allow my body to give out on me. I was too close to victory, and so determined not to give up.

In September 2008, I won a title coveted by many ballroom dancing competitors. I became the United States Pro Am American Smooth DanceSport Champion in the thirty-five to fifty age group. At age fifty, I was elated to be able to pull off this victory with my declining left leg. At the time of my performance, I was blessed with being unaware of the detail of my leg issues.

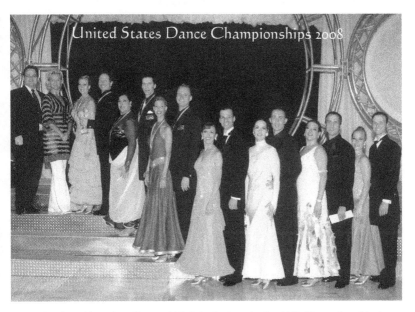

My husband/teacher Jim and I felt lucky to win the U.S. Championship in 2008 despite my severely damaged left hip joint

My husband, teacher, and dance partner, Jim Maranto, used his professional skills to masterfully choreograph my dance routines to accommodate and disguise my weak left leg. Retired from professional competition, Jim had changed his focus to teaching and competing with his many amateur students of all ages, shapes, sizes, and skill levels.

Jim, considered a master at Pro Am competition dancing, was able to minimize my weaknesses and showcase my strengths. I feel certain that not one person in the audience, nor one on the judging panel, was aware that I was dancing on a severely compromised left hip joint. In fact, at the time, none of us were aware of the severity of my hip situation.

A few months later, I came to the conclusion that my chiropractic plan was neither alleviating my pain nor bringing me a reasonable solution to my problem. I began to feel depressed and lost again. I felt like I was being misled and not receiving proper counsel, so I made an appointment with an orthopedic doctor. This was definitely a step in the right direction, and certainly one I wish that I had made months earlier.

My hip X-ray painted a very clear picture and confirmed all of my suspicions. My left hip joint had little-to-no cartilage, and was thus bone on bone. Ouch! In spite of my bleak situation, this doctor advised me to put off surgery because at age fifty-one, I was considered too young for a hip replacement. I was frightened when the doctor told me that a new hip joint might last for only ten or fifteen years. Once again, I was feeling lost and unclear about how to proceed. The doctor advised me to try physical therapy in order to increase mobility in my hip joint. I was skeptical. Sure, I believed that my range of motion might improve, but what was going to kill my pain? *Hello! Is anyone hearing me? I am in pain! I am miserable!* Feeling as though I was running out of options, I reluctantly agreed to follow the doctor's advice.

My physical therapy sessions consisted of daily workouts on the stationary bike and the elliptical machine, along with a series of stretching exercises. Twice a week I would go for sessions of more intense assisted stretching by a physical therapist. Honestly, the program did improve my range of motion slightly; however, the joint pain was ever present and growing worse.

The orthopedic doctor had also advised me to take a daily anti-inflammatory drug called Feldene®, and steroid injections every six months along with Vicodin® to ease my pain while dancing. I was concerned about what damage these drugs might be doing to my body. The doctor advised me that taken as prescribed, and in moderation, the drugs would not cause me harm.

I had heard all kinds of wild stories about celebrities taking fists full of Vicodin® and becoming addicted to various painkillers. I told the doctor that I did not want to follow the *celebrity diva* path of drug rehab. He laughed and suggested that I start with one half of a Vicodin® to see how it worked for me.

Half of a Vicodin® did not do much at all for me. Actually, I did not even find one or two Vicodin® to be all that helpful. Nor did it make me feel crazy or drugged out in any way. Maybe if I had taken thirty or forty pills, like some of the celebrities I had heard about, then some real pain killing might have occurred. I was not willing to try that experiment. These "bandages" as I referred to the drugs and physical therapy, enabled me to keep dancing and competing for another five months. I finally reached the point where I realized that nothing was going to magically fix my hip. My depression was increasing and I felt like I was wasting time and money following this path of quick fixes and drugs. Unable to endure the increasing pain, my body forced me to quit dancing in mid-July 2009.

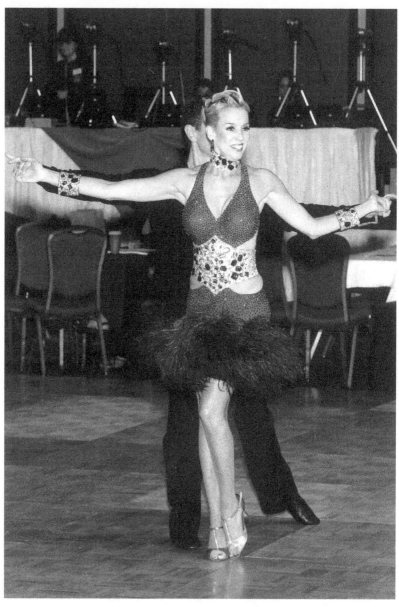

I had hoped that physical therapy and drugs would enable me to dance another year to defend my championship title. Unfortunately, my chronic pain forced me to quit dancing in July 2009.

## Patients in Pain

If you are experiencing chronic leg pain of any sort, whether it be in your groin area, your knee area, front of leg, or back of leg, do not go to a chiropractor, Rolfer, acupuncturist, or massage therapist for *diagnosis* of the problem. Go directly to the best orthopedic doctor you can find and ask for a hip X-ray.

## Chapter 2

# Dr. Wise

Stifling an urge to dance is bad for your health—
it rusts your spirit and your hips.

**—Terri Guillemets**

Chatting with my friend on the phone one day, I was bellyaching about not being able to dance anymore. My friend had her own hip related issues, and was able to commiserate with me. I was feeling so defeated and weary from all of the wasted time and money that I had spent on failed treatments and therapies.

I asked my friend, "Why do all of these doctors want to see me suffering? Why don't they tell me to get a hip replacement?"

After following my painful journey, my friend could sense my drained spirit and see that I was really in need of some guidance. She had been married to a physician, so she was able to ask for his assistance in seeking out advice on my behalf. Word came back to me that I should not make any hasty decisions about hip replacement surgery, but should first have a consultation with a particular doctor who was the former chairman of orthopedics at a large university hospital. No longer performing hip replacement surgeries, this doctor's skill and experience had inspired him to focus on research and patient consultation.

*Yes! Finally!* I thought. I felt as though I had just been told that I was being sent off to see the Wizard! If I could have jumped in the air and clicked my heels together, I would have done so, gleefully. I did not even mind that I had to mess around with getting a referral from my friend's physician husband, along with the hassle of numerous phone calls and faxes required to snag one of the coveted appointment times. I waited weeks for this meeting with the esteemed expert.

I had not danced for a month, and my nagging groin pain was increasing along with my depression. My daily gym workouts had diminished to a few minutes on the recumbent stationary bike and a few exercise machines where I could sit down and work my upper body. My spirits were elevated knowing that I was finally going to get advice and direction from a wise, highly respected, orthopedic expert. Feeling confident with this referral and recommendation by two well-respected doctors in town, I believed that my salvation was just around the corner. I was going to meet a wise man who would show me empathy and offer a solution to my pain. I believed that, like Dorothy, I was on my way to Oz to see the Wizard.

The day finally arrived, and I cheerfully hobbled into the wizard's office with X-ray in hand. After viewing my X-ray, the doctor came into the examining room to meet me. He offered a brief, bland introduction, and then he mumbled something about degeneration of joint cartilage. The "brilliant" doctor was not forthcoming with information, suggestions, or solutions, so I had to ask questions just to create some ongoing dialogue with this impersonal guy. Dr. Wise, as I will facetiously refer to him, was not sympathetic to my physical pain, much less my emotional pain.

As I lay on the examining table, Dr. Wise jerked my knee up to my chin, without warning, as I winced in pain. He mumbled something about my range of motion not being so good. *Duh,* I thought. Since I had just finished telling Dr. Wise about how much pain I was experiencing, one would think that he might have been a bit gentler.

"Should I get a hip replacement?" I asked him.

"You can if you want to," he replied.

I was extremely annoyed by Dr. Wise's trite response. This doctor, supposedly at the top of his field, had just seen my X-ray (which I already knew was bad) and he could not even give me a straight answer or an honest opinion? Like the other orthopedic doctor who I had seen, Dr. Wise went on to tell me that I was really quite young for a hip replacement, because they are not expected to last more than ten, or possibly fifteen years. *Hello! Do these guys really expect me to limp around, suffering in excruciating pain, wasting my life away for years before getting any relief?* It seemed as though these doctors were just giving me some standard, textbook answer, instead of addressing me as an individual patient.

Feeling agitated, I proceeded to ask Dr. Wise about a couple of surgeons who had been recommended to me, to which he responded, "Any one of them can do the surgery."

I was so angry at this point that I wanted to spit in his face. I had waited weeks to see this highly regarded doctor, who sees patients only on referral from illustrious colleagues, and he could not even be bothered to steer me in the right direction. Dorothy must have felt this way after her long, weary, journey to Oz when she found the Wizard of Oz to be an insensitive jerk. Feeling dejected, and just downright pissed at that point, I realized that the man behind this curtain was certainly no wizard, not in my opinion, based on this pathetic experience. The wise doctor would not even console me by recommending a good surgeon. We all know that some surgeons come highly recommended, and others not so much. Dr. Wise offered me nothing—no surgeon's name, no empathy, no encouragement, and no hope.

I pointed out to Dr. Wise that I wanted a surgeon who works with athletes; one who would help me to accomplish my goal of getting back to competitive ballroom dancing. Dr. Wise asked me to describe what, specifically, was required of one's body for dancing (apparently he had never seen or heard of ballroom dancing). I told him that I must be able to move with leg strength, power, and speed backwards down the floor in high heels, as well as swivel my hips and change direction rapidly at times.

Dr. Wise shook his head and responded, "You'll be able to walk again, but you will not be able to dance again."

I felt my blood pressure go up. I was biting my tongue. I informed Dr. Wise that I had several friends who are not only dancing, but also competing with their new hips and new knees.

Dr. Wise seemed a bit perplexed and did not have much of a response. One could easily surmise that this man had no knowledge or experience regarding athletes and joint replacement surgery.

I decided to throw one last question at Dr. Wise. I asked him if I should try "prolotherapy," which I had learned is the injection of a mixture including dextrose into the attachment point of the tendon or ligament on the bone. I had several friends who had heard that successful prolotherapy treatment eliminates pain and improves joint stability.

Dr. Wise offered that prolotherapy, used mostly for knees, is questionable, experimental, and not guaranteed to work. He suggested that the only way to find out if it would work for me would be to give it a try. My frustration and desperation prodded me to sign up for the prolotherapy treatment program.

I was shocked when I saw that the paperwork from Dr. Wise was for HYALGAN® injections[1]—something entirely different from

---

1    HYALGAN® is a registered trademark of Fidia Farmaceutici S.p.A., Italy, http://www.hyalgan.com.

prolotherapy! HYALGAN® is made from a natural, highly purified sodium hyaluronate that comes from rooster combs. Hyaluronate is a natural chemical in our bodies that acts as a lubricant and shock absorber in the joints. Osteoarthritis patients are lacking hyaluronate in their joint fluid and tissues.

Did Dr. Wise, the worldly researcher, not know about prolotherapy? Did he think that the two formulas were one and the same? Actually, I had read about the "rooster comb" injections, as well as the "sugar" injections, and as a last ditch effort, I was willing to try just about anything.

I knew in my heart that this new HYALGAN® treatment would probably not be a magic cure. In fact, the odds of it working at all were not even favorable. What does one do after numerous devastating failures? Give up? I could not just let my life dwindle away and continue to endure the pain and depression. I was yearning to find someone who would look me in the eye, tell me the truth, and help me! I so desperately wanted to meet a doctor, who could say to me, "I want to help you, I can help you, and I will help you." *Why does this have to be so damn difficult?* I thought.

Over the next month, I had a series of three HYALGAN® injections. I went to the hospital and lay on the table while a nice, young doctor injected my hip joint with a giant syringe of, as I liked to say, "rooster cartilage." Each time, I saw a different doctor and nurse. They were always intrigued to learn that they were treating a ballroom dancer. After hearing my story, all were sending me off with well wishes toward making it back to the competition floor to defend my United States title. I felt that even if this treatment was just another quick fix, if it would enable me to dance at the U.S. Championships in another few weeks, then it would be worth the hassle and the expense. The doctors had informed me that if the treatment was going to present positive results, I would not feel any relief until after the third injection.

Several weeks and three thousand dollars later, I hit rock bottom. The HYALGAN® injections had been unsuccessful. I was unable to dance at all; so competing and defending my title at the 2009 United States DanceSport Championships was sadly out of the question. Once again, I felt like Dorothy when she was on her way to Oz, and had no clue of which way to follow the yellow brick road. She saw the scarecrow hanging up there saying, "You could go this way, or that way, or both ways."

I had been traveling in circles, and I could find neither Oz, nor the Wizard. At that point I would have settled for a scarecrow, a tin man, or a lion. I needed a friend who knew my pain. I needed a friend who could help me find the yellow brick road and get me started on my way down the right path.

 DARLA'S TIPS FOR

### Patients Who are Seeking an Orthopedic Surgeon

1.  If you meet with a doctor who shows you no sympathy, and makes you feel insignificant to the point where you want to grab him around the throat and breathe fire into his face, then it is best to keep searching. You will eventually find a doctor who shows you kindness and has a true desire to help you.

2.  Seek out friends and acquaintances who have had hip replacement surgery. Patients love to praise a doctor who heals them and makes them feel good.

## Chapter 3

# What a Difference a Doctor Makes

Some men have thousands of reasons why they cannot do what they want to, when all they need is one reason why they can.

**—Martha Graham**

Having reached the point where I had exhausted all options in dealing with my hip pain, I was at an all-time emotional low. Everyone, from the Rolfer, to the chiropractor, to the physical therapist, to the orthopedic doctor, to the wise orthopedic master, had encouraged me to put off surgery. It had become painfully obvious to me that no therapies, treatments, nor drugs were going to magically build cartilage in my hip or erase my intense joint pain.

Faced with no longer being able to do my daily gym workouts, or participate in dance competitions, I felt as though I was losing important and special elements of my life. I did not want to live limping around in pain, day after day. I was both sad and outraged that the doctors did not seem to sympathize with my pain and dwindling quality of life. Why could they not understand how much I was hurting physically and emotionally? Why did they not want to take away my pain and make me happy again? Why did they think that I should suffer for ten more years before getting hip replacement surgery? Why could they not understand that I wanted to live and enjoy life in the present?

My friend Cecelia, a social dance teacher at Jim's Phoenix studio, had recently had hip replacement surgery. She seemed to be making steady progress, while I was wasting time on frivolous fixes, and enduring months of misery. Cecelia said that her surgeon seemed "pretty good" and "really nice," which were terms that I would never use to describe my recent experience with Dr. Wise. Cecelia referred me to Dr. Anthony Hedley at the Arizona Institute for Bone and Joint Disorders.

Around that same time, my friend Patricia told me that her renowned heart surgeon had had a hip replacement and returned to his work in the operating room nine days after the surgery. *That surgeon must be fabulous,* I thought. Having promised to get the name of her heart doctor's hip surgeon, one day Patricia handed me a piece of paper with the name Dr. Hedley written on it. *Aha! This Dr. Hedley is the same guy who did Cecelia's hip replacement surgery.* If a prominent heart surgeon chose this orthopedic surgeon to do his personal hip replacement, then this doctor had to be the best. I finally felt as though I were traveling down the correct path.

I was able to get an appointment with Dr. Hedley without having to pull strings, jump through hoops, or endure a long wait. Prior to my meeting with Dr. Hedley, the technician took a new X-ray of my hip, and his nurse took a detailed account of my history of misery.

Although my situation was dire, after viewing my X-ray, Dr. Hedley greeted me with a smile and offered sympathy. He propped his laptop up on the table with my X-ray in full view on the screen.

"How can someone as small as you have a hip that looks this bad?" he offered, with a caring expression of concern. It was bad news, but I felt comforted by his empathy and demeanor.

Dr. Hedley went over the picture with me, and pointed out the grim details. He showed me where there was no cartilage, and bone was actually touching bone. The hip joint consists of a ball and socket, and this socket was not sufficiently covering all of the bone. With great confidence, Dr. Hedley asserted, "You have no choice. You must get a hip replacement."

*Hallelujah!* I felt such relief and joy. Finally, a doctor who is not afraid to be honest. I had been searching so long for this kind smile, offering a solution to my pain and depression.

Again, with confidence and assurance, Dr. Hedley told me, "I'll fix your hip and have you dancing again in no time. You weigh 110 pounds? This will be so easy."

I think my smile grew brighter than Dr. Hedley's. This was the first time I limped out of a doctor's office with an ear-to-ear grin, along with feelings of comfort, joy, and confidence. That day I walked out of Dr. Hedley's office with a solution, a surgeon, a surgery date, and a smile. I had finally made it to Oz and met the Wizard!

Later that day I reflected back on my long journey. I had some disturbing thoughts and concerns regarding the doctors whom I had seen prior to meeting Dr. Hedley. When Dr. Hedley's nurse was checking me in and writing up my history, she had asked me about the location of my pain, as did all of my previous doctors. As always, I explained that my pain was at the top of my leg, in the crease, where the leg meets the body. I remember telling the nurse that my chiropractor had emphatically denied that this pain was caused from a bad hip.

She chuckled and shook her head as she told me, "Everyone knows that pain in the groin is a classic symptom of hip pain."

Could the chiropractor really not have known about a classic symptom of hip pain? *Hmmm....*

When my first orthopedic doctor viewed my X-ray, did he really not know that there was no hope for a hip without any cartilage and where there was bone on bone? Did he really think that I was going to be able to go on for ten or fifteen more years with physical therapy, drugs, and steroid injections?

Months later, when I had my encounter with Dr. Wise, why was he not just straightforward and honest with me after looking at my X-ray? Why did he not tell me that I was wasting time trying to fix a severely damaged hip that really needed to be replaced?

 DARLA'S TIPS FOR

### Doctors, Chiropractors, and Physical Therapists

1. When a patient comes to you presenting classic symptoms of hip pain, you should be able to recognize those symptoms and suggest that the patient get an X-ray of the hip.

2. When a patient presents a hip X-ray showing no cartilage and bone touching bone, please be honest with the patient and do not recommend drugs, injections, and therapies that are only going to prolong the patient's agony.

 DARLA'S TIPS FOR

### Future Hip Replacement Patients

1. If you have been struggling with pain in your groin area, along with pain that follows down your whole leg, get yourself to a doctor who will X-ray your hip joint.

2. If you have agonizing pain while reaching out to close your car door, find it painful to just stand for more than five or ten

seconds, do not want to go into a store unless you are able to hang onto a shopping cart, do not want to walk up steps, find that the recumbent bike is the only thing you can still do at the gym, and if your depression is increasing daily, then it may be time for you to get hip replacement surgery!

## Chapter 4

# The Hospital Experience

The journey between who you once were, and
who you are now becoming, is where the
dance of life really takes place.

**—Barbara De Angelis**

I never imagined that I would get a date for my hip replacement surgery so quickly after my initial appointment with Dr. Hedley. It had been only a month and a half since my first meeting with Dr. Hedley, and there I was, limping out of bed with gusto, and preparing myself to go to the hospital. I was so excited, thinking that in several hours, I would be waking up with a brand new titanium hip, and all of those miserable days of pain and depression would be behind me.

I had been online, looking up well-known people who had undergone hip replacement surgery. I had read about tennis great, Jimmy Connors, who was so fearful about getting his hip replaced that he kept chickening out, and turned his car around twice on his way to the hospital. Jimmy later admitted that after the procedure, he felt better than he had in years. That story really made me laugh. My feelings about getting hip replacement surgery were the exact opposite of Jimmy Connor's feelings. I could not wait to get to the hospital and jump on that operating table. If I could have had a parade with a marching band escort me to the hospital, I would have cheerfully lead the way. In my mind, I was skipping with joy down the yellow brick road, off to see the Wizard.

Once Jim and I arrived at the hospital, it took a couple of hours to get me checked in and then prepped for surgery. We were taken to the surgery waiting area, where there were several other patients waiting for last minute instructions and introductions to medical staff.

I remember a woman on the gurney across the room from me who was waiting to have gastric bypass surgery. Her nervousness was displayed in her incessant stream of chatter. She kept calling her anesthesiologist "Dude," and told him how scared she was about five or six times. Poor thing, I did sympathize with her, but she was funny, and provided entertainment for Jim and me as we waited. I was not feeling nervous, but I was feeling anxious to get my surgery over with at that point.

We met the anesthesiologist who explained his role in the whole procedure. Next, a nurse came to stick an IV needle in the back of my hand. After her third attempt to get the needle into a vein, she said that she would try just one more time. *Ouch!* All of that poking around was really hurting my hand.

"Why can't you just stick it in my arm? I asked her.

The nurse explained that the IV lines would be "in the way," because later I would need to bend my arms and pull myself up onto the walker, and the IV line in the hand was just easier to maneuver around. I felt as badly for the nurse as I did for my poor hand. The fourth attempt with the needle, proved to be successful for the nurse. I really did not like that needle being in my hand, not even a little bit. I was starting to feel anxious. I wanted it all to be over.

*Let's get this show on the road!* I thought. *Uh oh, was I going to start losing it because of my agitation over some stupid little needle in my hand? No! I am about to receive a great gift. Relax!*

Dr. Hedley walked in the room with that familiar, comforting smile, and came over to greet us. He introduced himself to Jim, and apologized for being slightly behind schedule. Dr. Hedley explained that he had just been working on "a revision" surgery, which had taken more time than he had expected. Apparently, when hip replacements get mucked up elsewhere, Dr. Hedley is the wizard who repairs the problems and mistakes. I felt at peace knowing that I was in the good hands of a great surgeon.

Dr. Hedley told us that my surgery would take only about an hour and a half, and he offered to call Jim as soon as it was over. He flicked his pen out of his pocket, picked up his knee, and wrote Jim's phone number down, right there on the pant leg of his scrubs. *Now that's how not to lose a phone number. He's one cool Dude*, I thought.

Dr. Hedley told us that he had done over five thousand hip replacement surgeries at St. Luke's Hospital, and assured us that everything was going to go great. Some surgeries present more of a challenge for a surgeon, if, for instance, the patient is large and overweight, or there has been a traumatic injury to the hip. Dr. Hedley knew his craft, and his confidence assured us that he anticipated that my surgery would be a piece of cake. Dr. Hedley told me that he would see me in a few minutes. Jim went off to work feeling excited about seeing me with my new hip in a few hours.

Next thing I knew, I was being wheeled on my gurney, down long hallways, onto an elevator, and out into another large room. The anesthesiologist came over and explained to me that he was going to put a needle in my back, and I would soon be falling asleep. I do not remember anything after that, until I opened my eyes, and I was lying on the gurney, in the same place, in that same room.

"Are you taking me into surgery now?" I asked a nurse who was standing nearby.

"You're done!" she said.

"You're kidding. Really?" Surprised, I reached down and felt my bandaged hip area.

I looked at the nurse and said, "Wow, I feel fine; I'm ready to go home."

"No, you can't go home yet," she chuckled.

Soon after that I was wheeled back to my hospital room, where I would be spending the next two days. No doubt about it, my hip was quite sore, but it was a new hip, and I was excited for my future with this precious gift. One of the nurses hooked me up to some IV lines, one of which was a controlled morphine drip. I was able to push the release button as I desired, however, there was a limit to how much juice was dispersed within a period of time.

As promised, Jim got a phone call from Dr. Hedley, at the exact time predicted, with word that my surgery had gone perfectly. About an hour later, Jim and our friend, Vonnie came in for a visit with me. Both were surprised to find me in good spirits and not whacked out by the experience or the medication. Knowing of my affection for butterflies, Vonnie brought me two beautiful pink and brown magnetic butterflies, which she stuck to the metal bed frame. I thought to myself, *Like those butterflies, I will soon be flying across the dance floor....*

Honestly, looking back, the whole surgery experience was not so bad. There are just a few unpleasant situations that one has to endure as a patient in a hospital. The best thing to do is to accept them and bite the bullet, knowing that in three days you will be out of there, and on the fabulous yellow brick road to recovery. I did not enjoy having the IV stuck in my hand for three days, and having various solutions injected into the tubes periodically. Nor did I enjoy using a bedpan once or twice during those first twenty-four hours after surgery. Trying to sit up, get out of bed, onto the walker, into the bathroom, and onto the raised toilet seat was another painful challenge. Sometimes I would have to wake up in the middle of the night so that the nurses could check my blood pressure or temperature, and give me some medication.

The morphine was not a miracle worker for me, and I had no energy or desire to get up and out of bed. When the nurses did get me out of bed for my first spin down the hall on my walker, they warned me that I might feel a bit nauseous due to the anesthesia and medication that was in my body. I did not feel sick at all, but I did feel something. It felt as though a giant shark was biting my butt and it just would not let go. *Ouch*!

My walker and I slowly shuffled down the halls, and around past the nurses' station a couple of times. Jim walked beside me that first day. It was nice to have him there with me, because I was feeling lethargic and unmotivated. Two laps around felt like quite enough for one day. I got back to my room, and with Jim's assistance, maneuvered myself off of my walker and into a chair. Seconds later, along came the nausea. I usually have a very tolerant stomach, and I almost never get sick from food that I have eaten. This sudden nausea was alarming, and I knew that I was about to lose it.

I looked up at Jim and said, "I think I'm going to be sick."

Luckily Jim sensed that time was of the essence, and he was able to sprint to the nurses' station, and get back with a pink bucket just in time, without a second to spare. *Ugh*. I did not feel so well, but I felt like the worst was behind me, and I was ready to move forward and face new challenges.

There were a variety of food choices offered to me in the hospital, and some even looked pretty good, however my usual healthy appetite was on hiatus. The morning after my surgery, Jim showed up to visit me with one of my most favorite things in hand: A Starbucks tall, double shot, two pump, soy mocha. Anyone who knows me knows that this small drink is the highlight of each and every one of my days. It is something that I always look forward to and never grow tired of—to the point where it always leaves me wanting more. Jim set the drink down on the tray in front of me. I looked at my all-time favorite soy mocha and felt absolutely no desire for it. *What's wrong with me? This is serious,* I thought with concern. Something had to be really wrong for me to lose the desire for my Starbucks.

Jim was shocked to see me rejecting soy mocha. He knew that there was one other drink, which even topped the coffee drink on my favorites list. Jim really had the nurses laughing when he asked if he could bring me my other favorite drink—Chardonnay. Now, that's what I call love. The answer from the nurses was an emphatic "NO!"

Prior to beginning actual physical therapy exercises, I had to learn how to use my walker to go up and down steps, as well as to position myself to get in and out of a car. In addition, I had to learn to use my hip "tools" to put on pants, socks, and shoes without bending over.

The first exercises I did were very simple and were done right in my hospital bed. A few of them were ankle pumps, heel slides, gluteal squeezes, and short arc quads. The last thing I felt like doing was getting my swollen hip into a bathing suit and doing pool therapy two days after surgery. This was nothing strenuous, but I was lacking the energy and motivation to exercise. The therapist had me do simple things like walking forward, backward, and sideways, along with raising my knees and swinging my arms.

It did feel good to be able to move freely and fluidly in that water, as opposed to the small, choppy, steps that I had been taking on the walker. When it was over, I was glad that I had experienced the pool therapy. It was a positive experience for both my mind and my body. Making it through each simple therapy session was another baby step down the road to recovery.

Finally, I was sent home with my "hip precautions," which are the golden rules that all hip replacement recipients must obey. There are nine things one must never do, as well as nine things that one must always remember. For weeks, I lived in fear of breaking one of these "rules," and causing the unthinkable. I had heard stories about people who had inadvertently crossed their legs, and popped their new hip out of joint! The thought of making a mistake always left me feeling a bit on edge, so I carried the following list around with me and treated it like a coveted bible.

**St. Luke's Medical Center**
**Physical Therapy Department**
**Total Hip Replacement**
**Dos and Don'ts**

## Do Nots

1. DO NOT sit in any low, soft chair or stool, which requires bending the hips beyond a right angle (90 degrees) to either sit or stand—keep the knee below the hip. AVOID couches and recliners. LIMIT your sitting to 45-60 minutes at a time to prevent stiffness.
2. DO NOT sit in bucket seats in a car without pillows.
3. DO NOT sit on a toilet without an elevated toilet seat. Use "handicapped" public bathroom stalls.
4. DO NOT lean over to tie shoelaces, put on stockings, apply your underwear, or pick up objects from the floor.
5. DO NOT lie on your good side without two pillows between your legs (only if you have been given clearance by your doctor or have been instructed), and you have someone to help you log roll as shown in the hospital.
6. DO NOT bring your legs together or cross the midline.

7. DO NOT cross your knees or ankles.

8. If you are allowed to weight bear on your surgical leg, be cautious NOT to pivot on that extremity when standing and turning. Instead, walk your feet around by small steps.

9. Sit down carefully! DO NOT twist to one side to reach for the arm of a chair or your bed. This will result in a twisting motion at your hip.

## Dos

1. DO use your ambulation aid (crutches, walker, etc., and correct weight bearing) AT ALL TIMES, until your doctor tells you otherwise at your six-week check-up appointment.

2. DO keep your leg turned out in a neutral position (toes to ceiling) when you are sitting, lying in bed, or walking. Keep your legs apart at all times. (Use a pillow or wedge between your legs as a reminder.)

3. DO try to use chairs with arms to aid your rising to a standing position.

4. DO get in and out of bed the way you were shown by the physical therapist in the hospital.

5. DO your exercises daily as instructed. DO NOT use weights on your leg.

6. DO NOTIFY YOUR DOCTOR IMMEDIATELY if you experience severe pain in your hip or inability to bear weight on your leg.

7. DO make sure family/friends are aware of your hip precautions also, so they can help you to remember.

8. DO use cold packs (twenty minutes at a time) if you notice increased swelling in your hip/thigh.

9. DO call your PHYSICAL THERAPY DEPARTMENT with any questions regarding your hip.

Prior to leaving the hospital, I rehearsed going up and down steps, as well as getting in and out of a car. Finally, I was in a wheelchair, riding down the hospital elevator. Discharge! At last. Out of the wheelchair, onto the walker, into the car, and off we drove.

 **DARLA'S TIPS FOR**

## Hospital Patients

1. You are not going to feel great while you are in the hospital, but remember it is only a few days. Just suck it up and endure the minor pokes and prodding. Remember, you have received a precious gift—a brand new hip. The pain will soon be gone and you will be joyfully skipping down the yellow brick road of recovery.

2. A friend of mine who already had one hip replacement asked to be catheterized for her second surgery. This makes it so much more comfortable for the patient. No bedpan or painful struggling to get up out of bed, and to the restroom in the middle of the night. I wish that I had thought to ask to be catheterized.

## Chapter 5

# Rehab: The Key to the Speed and Quality of Recovery

Character cannot be developed in ease and quiet. Only through experience of trial and suffering can the soul be strengthened, ambition inspired, and success achieved.

**—Helen Keller**

After leaving the hospital, I found my first week to be challenging, and somewhat painful, yet I was ready to take it all on and move forward with my recovery. My hip was really swollen, which was alarming to Jim. I was aware that my hip was somewhat bigger, however I had not looked very closely at it, as I was more worried about just getting around, and remembering important details required for my basic movements and actions.

On the first day after my release from the hospital, I was anxious to wear my normal clothing and resume my life. Implementing my new hip tool, I squeezed the handle to open the pincer type mechanism at the end of the long stick. Without bending over, I picked up a pair of my cute Capri jeans to put on, which caused Jim to burst out laughing.

"Darla, you're not going to get into those!" he exclaimed.

I guess looking down from my angle, my hip did not appear to be gigantic, but apparently it was exactly that and more. I do not know why I thought I could get those tight jeans up over my big fat hip. We had a good laugh over that one. Fortunately for me, leggings and sweatpants were in style. My hip was fine and everything appeared to be progressing normally, as was confirmed by my homecare nurse who stopped by a couple of times that first week.

I did not really focus much on the size of my hip, as I had other more important things on my mind. I was concerned about cleaning and dressing my wound, taking the correct amount of medications at the right times, getting in and out of the bathroom and shower with my walker, dealing with my hip tools, and following the feared hip precautions. I was almost haunted by the thought that I might inadvertently break one of "the rules." If I thought that I was forgetting something, I would pull out the sheet of paper and read the part in question, such as: *Do keep your leg turned out in a neutral position (toes to ceiling) when you are sitting, lying in bed, or walking. Keep your legs apart at all times. (Use a pillow or wedge between your legs as a reminder.)*

The other rule that worried me was the one that said: *When bearing weight on your surgical leg, be cautious not to pivot on that extremity when standing and turning. Instead, walk your feet around by small steps.*

Yikes, all of those demands made me so nervous. My dancing life is full of swivels and pivots. I even had to think in advance of sitting on furniture or car seats in order to avoid a situation where my knee was higher than my hip. The angle between my torso and thighs was not permitted to exceed ninety degrees in any position. I could sit on a chair with arms, and a firm seat, or use pillows to create the proper angle. In addition, I had to always be aware of maintaining an eighteen-inch space between my legs. So many things to remember, and I thought some of my dance routines were a challenge to the memory!

I thought that I would go crazy sleeping on my back without moving to another position all night long. I had a pillow wedged between my knees to prevent me from crossing my legs, however not being able to roll over onto one side or the other, was making me feel like I was in a straitjacket. In the hospital, one of the therapists had shown me how to do the "log roll," which permitted me to put a pillow between my legs, and roll over onto my right side. I was terrified to try this "log roll" for the first time for fear that I would do something detrimental to my new hip. I had to do it for my sanity. I was not allowed to roll over on my new left hip, but at least I could move freely from sleeping on my back to my right side as many times as I desired throughout each night.

It was challenge learning to use the hip tools to put on pants and socks. I had to wear these ugly, white, surgical stockings for six weeks, and it was tough getting them on without bending over and breaking that ninety-degree rule. I was allowed to go without the stockings for only one-to-two hours per day. Sometimes I just wanted to scream, rip them off, and toss them in the trash. Nevertheless, I wore them faithfully, out of fear, knowing that they were important in reducing swelling, and promoting good circulation. I did not want to get a blood clot.

Since Jim was working all hours of the day, my friend, Debbie, came to visit and keep me company for my first two days out of the hospital, and then Jim's mom spent the next few days with me. Always on my walker, we went on two walks per day. The hip pain was still there, yet somewhat diminished. Instead of feeling like a great white shark was biting my butt, it felt like the bite of a tiger shark or a bull shark.

Once again, I was gung ho for my daily Starbucks fix, and my appetite was slowly returning. Like old times, I found myself looking forward to dinnertime and a Chardonnay. I became so adept with my walker that I was able to go to a restaurant and a movie theater. I was so happy to be out, that I did not care if people were staring at me with my walker.

I continued my home exercise program with supervision from a physical therapist, once a week, for about a month. I was still sore, and fatigued, so we cautiously and slowly added to my assortment of exercises. On the bed, I could do side-lying leg lifts, bridges (lifting my butt up off the bed), and straight leg raises. Eventually I even added ankle weights as I did my long arc quads, sitting at the side of the bed. I knew that ankle weights were forbidden on the hip precautions list, however these were very light, and recommended by my home therapist. Standing at a countertop, I could do mini squats, and heel raises, along with some side and back leg lifts.

Finally it was time to give up the walker and practice walking around the house solo. I was feeling fearful at first, and my therapist pointed out that I was not even walking properly. I had to concentrate on taking equally sized steps, and bearing weight evenly on both legs. I continued to use a cane both in the house, and in public, for a couple more weeks after giving up the walker. I did not want to risk stumbling or falling.

My goal was to keep making baby steps of progress with my baby steps of therapy. I still had pain and fatigue for the first few weeks after surgery, and my progress was slow. There I was, just trying to walk normally again and get through some simple exercises each day. With most of my time spent indoors, I found myself feeling depressed as I thought about the long road ahead of me. I recalled Dr. Wise's annoying words to me: *"You will be able to walk again, but you will not be able to dance."*

What if Dr. Wise was right? What if this new hip was not going to give me the power that I needed to dance at the top level? I did not want to accept that there was even a slim possibility that that could be true. I wanted to prove that Dr. Wise was wrong. I wanted to make it back to the competition floor, and not be just an okay dancer, or even a pretty good dancer; I wanted to be an excellent dancer, and a champion— perhaps the first champion ever with an artificial hip.

About three weeks after my surgery, I was excited to go as a spectator with Jim and his students to one of the biggest competitions of the year—The Ohio Star Ball. A friend cautioned me that perhaps I might not want to be seen by my competitors, or judges, in my injured state. Did I want them to see me using a cane, and admitting to having had major joint replacement surgery? There is something to be said about not allowing the opposition, and the judges, to see you when you are not fit and strong. Perhaps they would develop negative thoughts, which could influence future reflections regarding my abilities.

One thing I learned when I studied sports psychology is that people do not tend to remember an athlete's times of failure or weakness. It is the great performances and victories that are always remembered. And everyone cherishes a great comeback story. I likened myself to the legendary racehorse, Seabiscuit, and his jockey Red Pollard. People had written them off as both recuperated from severe injuries. It was doubtful that either one of them would recover and return to racing. Seabiscuit and Red came back against the odds to win the Santa Anita Handicap in 1940, laying down the second-fastest mile-and-a-quarter time in American racing history. *Seabiscuit came back and ran to victory, and I will come back and dance to victory.*

As I meandered around the Ohio Star Ball competition on my cane, I bumped into one of my friendly competitors. Her eyes filled with tears, as she must have imagined the worst for me at first sight. Her unexpected, authentic concern warmed my heart, as much as it shocked me.

I found myself comforting my friend, telling her, "No, I'm fine! I just got a new hip. It's titanium. I've got an unfair advantage now. I'm going to come back soon and beat the pants off of everybody!"

I did not want people to feel sorry for me. I wanted everyone to jump on the bandwagon with me and travel joyously down my road of recovery.

I began to wonder if there was athlete with an artificial hip who had ever come back to win a U.S. championship in any sport. I had heard of a few professional athletes who had come back to participate successfully in their sports with their new hips, but had any of them won a major championship?

My curiosity led me to stumble across the story of John Wensich. The competitive bodybuilding, power lifting, running, and martial arts training since the 1960s had taken a toll on John's body. Along with broken bones and ribs, John developed a serious case of osteoarthritis. He had one hip replacement in 1990, and another one done in 1991. After ten years, those hip implants wore out, and John had two additional hip replacement surgeries in 2000 and 2002. Citing rehabilitation as the key element to his recovery, John had a stellar competition season in 2007. He won the United States Bodybuilding Federation North American Championships over-fifty-five class, the Natural Physique Association Universe over-sixty class, and the National Gym Association national bodybuilding competition in the over-sixty division. John Wensich competed and won against people who had no arthritis, and never had surgery. He won after having four hip replacements! *Wow, that is something! I want to achieve greatness like that.*

Perhaps John Wensich was the first athlete with an artificial hip to win a United States championship. A great accomplishment, yes, but he did not have to run backwards down the dance floor, with speed and power in two-and-a-half-inch high heels! Bodybuilding did not require any swift, traveling movement. A bodybuilder does not have to take more than a few steps in a routine.

I continued to wonder if there had ever been a baseball player, a basketball player, a football player, a hockey player, a tennis player, a golfer, or a dancer who had won a major national championship after having hip replacement surgery?

Could I possibly come back from this surgery and become the first athlete, with an artificial hip, to win a United States championship in a sport that required traveling movement? I was having difficulty merely walking properly, unassisted by my cane, and there I was thinking that I could come back and dance my way to a United States championship title. Ha! Was I crazy or what?

It was times like that, when I really wished that my mother and father were still alive. I really wanted to talk to them. I thought to myself, *what would they say?* My mother probably would not have known if she should encourage me to have such a lofty goal. She herself had had a hip replacement and never did much other than walk afterward.

I felt certain that I knew exactly what my father would say to me. He would recite his favorite quote by Fred Van Amburgh: "Dream big dreams, then put on your overalls and go out and make the dreams come true." Okay then, that is what I will do, I decided. I will pull my overalls up over this big, fat hip, and go out to the field, and start farming my dreams.

 **DARLA'S TIPS FOR**

## The Recovering Patient

1. You will feel fatigued, weak, and sore for a couple of weeks after surgery. Rome was not built in a day, so do not expect too much too soon. It is okay to have a big goal, but be realistic and know that recovery and rehabilitation take time and work.

2. Do your therapy exercises every day. You might not feel motivated, and the exercises are likely to appear simple and trite, however these small steps will be the building blocks of your future stability and success.

3.  Keep a positive, upbeat mental attitude. You will not be permitted to drive a car for six weeks, so rely on friends and family members to take you out and about.

## Chapter 6

# Setting a Realistic and Safe Goal after Hip Replacement Surgery

> You have to do what others won't
> to achieve what others don't.
>
> **—Anonymous**

There has been explosive growth in the number of joint replacement surgeries performed worldwide over the past few decades. Originally, the purpose of a total hip replacement was to relieve pain experienced in everyday activities. Years ago, patients were primarily elderly with non-active lifestyles. They were not expected to outlive the fifteen-to-twenty-year lifetime of a new hip implant. The only goal these hip replacement patients had was to be able to walk and sleep comfortably, get up and down steps, and be able to put on shoes and socks.

New advances in surgery have made hip replacements enticing for a younger population. Hoping for more than merely pain relief, younger hip replacement patients expect to resume an active, athletic lifestyle, and some seek to return to sports activity that is perceived to be unrealistic and unsafe. Harsh physical demands on a new implant can affect its durability and lifespan.

Medical professionals want to encourage hip replacement recipients to pursue healthy lifestyles. At the same time, patients should be cautioned to avoid certain types of exercise. There are recommendations, but there are no real validated guidelines on accepted activities after hip replacement surgery. How much activity and impact can a hip implant take? What sports are safe, and how aggressively can an athlete participate in a sport? A weekend athlete and a highly competitive athlete have different goals, along with vastly different levels of intensity.

Studies have shown that high-impact sports such as rugby, football, hockey, and basketball bring a high risk of traumatic complications, including dislocation and fracture around the prosthesis. On the other end of the spectrum, a sedate round of golf is unlikely to cause serious harm. Ice-skating is considered a safe activity, while hockey is considered unsafe due to the heavy contact interaction of the athletes.

An experienced athlete returning to water skiing or surfing brings skills that will minimize his risk, whereas a beginner attempting such sports for the first time might be putting himself in jeopardy. Yoga and Pilates can be resumed with avoidance of positions that extend beyond traditional, posterior hip precautions. Martial arts can be resumed, but patients must avoid sparring and high kicks.

Running and jogging after hip replacement surgery is a concern due to the duration of repetitive load on the joint—it takes five times the body weight with each heel strike. Running short distances infrequently, as in doubles tennis or softball, is less stressful and considered acceptable and safe movement. Low impact alternatives are encouraged for maintaining cardio-vascular fitness. These include: power walking, biking, and swimming, as well as use of the stair climber and elliptical machines.

I came across the Hip Society's detailed table of sports activities recommended for hip replacement patients.

## Recommended/Allowed Sports

| | |
|---|---|
| Stationary bicycling | Low-impact aerobics* |
| Croquet | Road cycling* |
| Ballroom dancing | Bowling* |
| Golf | Canoeing* |
| Horseshoes | Hiking* |
| Shooting | Horseback riding* |
| Swimming | Cross-country skiing* |
| Doubles tennis | |
| Walking | |

*\* Recommended only to experienced athletes*

## Not Recommended

| | |
|---|---|
| High-impact aerobics | Jogging |
| Baseball/softball | Lacrosse |
| Football | Racquetball |
| Gymnastics | Rock climbing |
| Handball | Squash |
| Hockey | Soccer |
| Singles tennis | Volleyball |

## No Conclusion

| | |
|---|---|
| Jazz dancing | Rowing |
| Square dancing | Speed walking |
| Fencing | Downhill skiing |
| Ice-skating | Weight lifting |
| Roller/inline skating | |

After studying this list, I noticed that ballroom dancing was on the recommended list, which is great; however, I feel certain that the members of the Hip Society who compiled this list might not have a full understanding of high-level ballroom dancing. They probably view ballroom dancing as meandering and shuffling around the dance floor at a country club dance or wedding.

The kind of high-level ballroom dancing that I aspired to return to came pretty close to high-impact aerobics, running, and jazz dancing, which were not on the Hip Society's recommended list. Of further concern is that ballroom dancing is not without jolting collisions on the competition floor from time to time. Unfortunately, not all male dancers are skilled at "floor craft." Yikes!

Was I crazy to think that I could come back after hip replacement surgery and dance my best ever? Could I go so far as to believe that I could become a U.S. champion in my highly contested Pro Am category with this new hip? The fact is that studies are unclear as to how far a patient can safely test the limits of a hip replacement. I suppose this is why some doctors hesitate to encourage involvement in sports after hip surgery. The possible consequences associated with a sports mishap are terrifying to contemplate. After going through all of the pain and agony preceding this precious gift of a new hip, who wants to risk allowing it to get worn out, loosened, dislocated, or fractured? Many athletes return to a sport ignoring their surgeon's recommendations and warnings. Some surgeons have worked more closely with athletes, thus have greater knowledge and ability to counsel patients who are athletically inclined. A patient's expectations and desire to compete in sports will have an influence on a surgeon's implant choice and surgical technique. Obviously, Dr. Wise did not know diddly-squat about an athlete's potential to return to sports activity.

## Goal-Setting with Your New Hip

1. Patients need to be aware of the risks involved with participation in sporting activities after hip replacement surgery.

2. Current literature does not answer the question as to whether it is safe for you to return to sports after a hip replacement, and orthopedic surgeons offer varying opinions as to which activities are recommended, and those that are not. Therefore, it will be most beneficial to seek out an experienced surgeon who has worked with many athletes.

3. Some patients recover more fully than others, therefore the decision to return to athletic activity should be guided by your surgeon and your physical therapist.

## Chapter 7

# Tom Watson Gave Me Hope and Inspiration

*In the midst of winter, I finally learned that there was in me an invincible summer.*

**—A. Camus**

As I continued to make baby steps of progress with my rehabilitation, I was feeling pleased overall. Nevertheless, doubts would sometimes try to creep into my mind and mess with my optimism. I would often have to give myself pep talks. I reminded myself that only four months ago, I was miserable with pain and emotionally defeated.

I reflected back to the last time I had danced. It was at the 2009 Virginia State Championships. I was able to produce a good result by placing second in my big event, however, I was really miserable. In spite of the medication, my hip was sore and both of my legs were hurting from top to bottom. It was so uncomfortable for me to just stand still in one place for more than two seconds in those heels. I knew that I could not go on like that anymore. I was so depressed and yearning for someone to tell me that my leg was going to soon be fixed, relieving me of all of my pain. I needed something—a sign—something to encourage me, something to pull me out of the dark hole.

Winding down after a long day of dancing at the competition, my golf enthusiast husband flipped on the television in our hotel room. Lo and behold, there it was…exactly what I needed…an inspiration…the remarkable Tom Watson. At fifty-nine years old, this hip replacement patient was tied for the lead of the prestigious British Open Golf Tournament.

"Are you kidding me?" I enthusiastically questioned Jim.

I needed to know how something as wonderful as this could come about, so I flipped open my laptop and got all the answers.

After a lifelong career of professional golf and victories in eight major championships, hip pain was making the sport unbearable for Tom Watson. In spite of the pain, Watson still had two wins, and four top ten finishes on the Champions Tour in 2008. I felt such a connection with Watson's story, as I too had pushed through my pain in 2008 to win my U.S. Championship title. Watson said the sharp pain prevented him from sleeping and reaching down to put on his socks and shoes.

*I sure knew what that felt like; shoes and socks are tough, yes, but try to paint your toenails. Ugh! That is painful.*

Watson felt like he could no longer play competitive golf due to his limited and dwindling range of motion. As I read more of Tom Watson's experience with his hip, it was like reading my own life story. Tom and I had identical reactions to our similar situations. Watson realized he was at the point where no therapy, exercise, or medication was going to remedy the situation. He just wanted it to be over as he said, "Let's get this done." I felt as though I was right there with Watson at that moment of realization. I could feel his emotion at that moment of surrender. I knew what it felt like to get to that point of giving up, and at the same time hoping for a brighter future.

Watson had commented, "This will be the first surgery I've had in my life. The only reason I'm doing it is to get rid of the pain. It's a quality of life decision. Fortunately, the medical world knows how to do this procedure very well. They have a great track record."

At age fifty-nine, Watson had thought that he probably could have made it another year on his bad hip, but the demands of tournament play exacerbated the pain. Of course, when he was not walking the course and swinging the club, his pain level went down. Since Watson still wanted to continue to play competitive golf, he felt that he just could not afford to put off surgery any longer.

Three months after total hip replacement surgery, Tom Watson resumed professional tournament golf. *Wow,* I thought. Three months sounded like such a short time of recovery and rehabilitation. Watson was not required to run fast, or leap through the air on his new hip, but still, three months sounded like no time at all to me.

Watson had won his first British Open title in 1975, the year Tiger Woods was born. It was thirty-four years later, nine months after his hip replacement surgery, and there was Watson at age fifty-nine, tied for the lead in regulation play of the 2009 British Open. It is impressive that an athlete of advanced age with an artificial joint could successfully compete at the top level of professional sports. Watson ended up losing the title to thirty-six year old Stuart Cink in a four-hole playoff. This was a heart-breaking loss for Watson, as he was so close to pulling off one of the most miraculous sporting achievements of all time.

Tom Watson did not win the big title that day, but he still left me in awe and inspired. A fifty-nine year old guy with a hip replacement was so close to being the oldest major championship winner ever!

This really got me to thinking. *Maybe I can achieve greatness with my new hip when I get it. Maybe I can be the first ballroom dancer with an artificial joint to win a U.S. Championship title. Yes, I can.*

Seeing Tom Watson's performance in that 2009 British Open golf tournament, planted a seed in my soul. Once again, I reflected back on my Dad's favorite quote: "Dream big dreams. Then put on your overalls."

## Chapter 8

# If Bo Jackson Can Run the Bases, Can I Run Down the Dance Floor in High Heels?

*If you believe in yourself, have dedication and pride and never quit, you'll be a winner. The price of victory is high, but so are the rewards.*

**—Paul Bryant**

My mind would drift off to deep thoughts as I muddled through my daily rehab exercises. Would I be completely pain-free in another couple of weeks? Would my new hip be strong and able to support my body while moving across the dance floor? Would my dancing get better, or would it be worse? Would people look at me and think, *Oh poor Darla, she looks weak and shaky.*

I needed to know what other athletes had experienced. Many athletes come back to participate in sports socially after hip replacement surgery. I've heard favorable testimonies of people who get along fine in their country club games of tennis and golf. Some well-known athletes have come back to give fine and memorable exhibition performances.

Other than Tom Watson, how many pro athletes have come back after hip replacement surgery to compete at the top of their game? Was there a pro athlete out there who had triumphed and achieved victory with an artificial hip? I needed to know if any such athletes existed. More importantly, had any of these athletes come back to participate in a sport that required running, or at least rapid, traveling movement? I needed a mentor—someone who's story I could cling to as a positive influence for my outlook on my own future.

My Internet searches quickly produced the name of the athlete who had a story that I was yearning to hear: Bo Jackson. Who would have thought that a two hundred twenty-five pound pro athlete, would turn out to be a major role model for a hundred and ten pound ballroom dancer? I was entranced as I read about Bo Jackson's athletic career.

Excelling in a sport is an aspiration of all serious athletes. Vincent "Bo" Jackson's unbelievable athletic ability earned him legendary status as a unique multi-sport athlete. Bo Jackson, one of the greatest running backs in National Football League history, simultaneously succeeded in pro baseball.

In high school, Jackson excelled in football, and baseball, as well as track and field. Collegiate recruiters in all three sports sought him out. Jackson's mesmerizing talent inspired the New York Yankees to draft the nineteen year old right out of high school in 1982. Wanting to pursue an education, Jackson rejected the multi-year contract, and accepted a football scholarship from Auburn. Jackson excelled as a college running back, and was awarded the prestigious Heisman Trophy, for the nation's most outstanding football player. This was quite an achievement, as Jackson considered the sport of football to be his hobby. The multi-talented Jackson continued to shine in college baseball, as well as track and field. He even gave some thought to joining the United States

Olympic team as a sprinter, however, was more drawn to the salary of an NFL player.

In 1986, both the National Football League's Tampa Bay Buccaneers, and Major League Baseball's Kansas City Royals drafted Jackson. Not wanting Jackson to become injured playing college baseball, the Buccaneers forced Jackson to choose between baseball and football. Jackson followed his heart and lifetime dream to be a major-league baseball player. Many were shocked as he turned down a five-year, $7.6 million football offer for a $1.06 million deal with the defending world champion Kansas City Royals. After spending most of the 1986 season in minor league baseball, the NFL's Los Angeles Raiders made Jackson a four-year contract offer, allowing him to continue to play baseball as well. In 1989, Jackson became the first athlete selected to play the All-Star Game of two major sports. He smacked a leadoff home run that earned him most valuable player status and led the American League to victory.

Jackson was named as an NFL All-Pro and in 1990 earned a selection to the Pro Bowl, an opportunity that he would never realize. Unfortunately, Jackson's football career ended January 13, 1991 when he suffered a serious hip injury while being tackled in a play-off game against the Cincinnati Bengals. The resulting condition, called Avascular Necrosis, was caused by decreased blood supply to the left femur. This led to deterioration of cartilage and bone around the hip joint.

After being released by the Royals in 1991, Jackson continued to try to play baseball, and signed with the Chicago White Sox. Making it through only twenty-three games, Jackson had to face the sad facts, and undergo hip replacement surgery.

I imagine that Bo Jackson, like the rest of us hip replacement prospects, must have felt the same sinking, hopeless feeling that we all know too well. We all try to stretch it out as long as possible with various treatments, therapies, and prayers. There comes a point where the body will just no longer respond to the valiant attempts at rehabilitation, and one must reluctantly surrender to the surgeon.

Medical and athletic experts assumed that Jackson's athletic career had ended. Jackson hated the painful and arduous rehabilitation process. Prior to his hip surgery, Jackson was so busy going back and forth from football to baseball, that he never made time for the gym workouts. Jackson hated the gym, which he thought was for wimps. Nonetheless, Jackson aggressively attacked his rehabilitation for the year following his surgery.

Back in shape, Jackson returned to the Chicago White Sox in 1993. Fulfilling a promise to hit a home run for his mother on his first swing of his first time at-bat, Jackson hit a pinch-hit home run to right field. This was perhaps the greatest moment of Bo Jackson's entire athletic career. He proved to be a world-class athlete, even after hip replacement surgery. Jackson was named the American League Comeback Player of the Year. In addition, he won the Tony Conigliaro Award, which is given to "a player who best overcomes an obstacle and adversity through the attributes of spirit, determination, and courage." The following year Jackson played with the California Angels batting a career high of .279. Sadly, Jackson's comeback was short-lived, as continuing knee problems forced him to retire from pro sports in 1995.

Bo Jackson's story gave me comfort and inspiration. If he could throw his hips into a home run hit, and run around the bases, then certainly, I could move from leg to leg, with power and speed across the dance floor. Bo Jackson made me believe in myself. He gave me the courage to embrace my hip replacement surgery, and look forward to great things to come.

## Chapter 9

# Rudy Galindo Skates with Two New Hips

The difference between the impossible and the possible
lies in a man's determination.

**—Tommy Lasorda**

I wanted to believe that I could achieve athletic victory with my new hip. During the initial weeks following my surgery, it was difficult at times to project my big positive picture of the future while I shuffled around with a cane and did those stupid, little exercises. In a quest for more inspiration, I curiously continued to research famous athletes who had returned to their sports after having total hip replacement surgery.

Rudy Galindo's story was particularly inspirational to me. I remember sitting mesmerized in front of my television, as Rudy astounded the figure skating world to win the 1996 Men's National Figure Skating Championship. My memories of that moment are so vivid. That was one of those special heart-warming experiences, watching an underdog take the prize. Rudy had never medaled in the men's singles competition. He had given up on his dream of winning a national championship, and essentially retired prior to this event. As an openly gay, Mexican American, Rudy felt that he would never be able to gain the political favor of the judges. In spite of Galindo's superior performance, the judging panel could have easily weighted their marks in favor of America's reigning world champion, Todd Eldredge. Rudy's memorable performance was a standout, and he won the gold. As I watched the event unfold, I felt as though I was right there next to Rudy, taking in the joy of his unexpected victory.

As I progressed with my research, I found Rudy's experience to be similar to mine in that we both had painful, declining hips, while still trying to squeeze out a few more performances. During 2001 and 2002, Rudy participated in a heavy season of exhibitions, including the strenuous Champions on Ice tour. He missed numerous performances due to an impending hip problem. Doctors diagnosed Galindo with AVN (Avascular Necrosis) a degenerative bone disease affecting both hips.

I read this quote from Rudy: "I was skating on dead bone, and it was deteriorating. It was painful. A doctor told me I would never skate again."

*Whoa*, I thought…*Déjà vu*. I recalled Dr. Wise's pessimistic words to me, "You will never dance again." The doctor's words seemed like a cruel, sharp, barb in the heart.

Rudy's skating career, and my dancing, both seemed terminated at the moment our doctors lowered the hatchet. In spite of disheartening news, there comes a point where one cannot endure excruciating hip pain any longer. Rudy was counseled to get both hips replaced. I can only imagine the fear that Rudy must have felt, facing two hip replacements, much less one.

Rudy's sister and coach, Laura, learned of the recently FDA approved ceramic on ceramic technique of total hip replacement. Thought to wear longer, and stay more secure than traditional plastic and metal implants, this surgery gave hope and promise to athletes. Rudy received two state-of-the-art ceramic hips only six weeks apart in the fall of 2003.

As most hip replacement patients are encouraged, Rudy began physical therapy immediately after surgery. I felt a kindred connection to Rudy when I heard his first feelings and descriptions regarding his new hip implants. He described the feeling of a bowling ball inside his hip. Rudy questioned how he would ever be able to do his jumps, with the sensation of heaviness. Conditioning and strengthening exercises for hours each day prepared Rudy to skate in The Champions on Ice tours that began in April 2004. Tom Collins, president of the tour, gushed over Rudy's remarkable return to the ice: "It's the most amazing thing I've ever seen from an athlete! It's unprecedented."

Once again, audiences watched Rudy perform his skillful jumps, including the salchow and double axle, as well as his shotgun spin. Learning of Rudy Galindo's comeback left me awestruck and inspired.

*If this guy can come back with two hip replacements, and show the courage, and strength to perform triple jumps through the air, landing his full body weight on one skinny little blade in a slippery ice rink, then I can certainly come back, with only one hip replaced, and dance on a stable wood floor!*

Thank you, Rudy! Thank you for giving me the fire and the desire! This kind of comeback would require from me the same amount of courage, heart, and perseverance that Rudy Galindo demonstrated. I believed that I had it in me. I was ready to begin my journey down the long yellow brick road to victory.

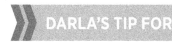

DARLA'S TIP FOR

## Choosing a Mentor

Search for people who share a similar plight with your experience and goals. Look at others who have achieved the unthinkable. Let the achievements of your mentors make you say to yourself, "If he could do that, then I can do this!"

## Chapter 10

# Wayne Sleep's New Hip Gets Him Back to the Royal Ballet

*It is not the size of a man*
*but the size of his heart that matters.*

**—Evander Holyfield**

It is odd to think that two people who are so extremely different and from different parts of the world, can end up being tied together with the common threads of life experiences. Several years ago, I would have scoffed at the mere suggestion that I could ever be writing a book. Even more unlikely would be the idea that one of the chapters in my book would be about a five-feet-two-inch tall, British, professional ballet dancer.

Here I am writing that book, while feeling a kindred connection to someone I never would have known about had we not shared common experiences of passion, pain, healing, and internal drive to recover, prove, and achieve.

Not too long ago, I hadn't heard of Wayne Sleep, and now I can say that Wayne Sleep has been both a mentor and a hero to me. We are two people who have never met, and it is unlikely that our paths will ever cross, but serendipitously, Wayne's life story has been a precious gift to me. Wayne's achievements have shown me what is possible and made me believe that I, too, could recover and thrive with a new hip. Wayne's story gave me the courage to pursue my own ultimate achievement. In learning of Wayne's battle through hip replacement surgery, and his impressive comeback to the Royal Ballet stage, I gained comfort and developed belief in the possibility of my own personal, future achievements. I became convinced that if Wayne Sleep could do what he did, then my dream of returning to top-level ballroom dance competition was possible as well. Seeing is believing. Dr. Wise took away my hope and my confidence in my dreams, but Wayne Sleep's heart-lifting story gave those things right back to me.

At five-feet-two inches tall, and several inches shorter than the required height of five feet eight inches, Wayne Sleep was the shortest person ever accepted into the Royal Ballet. In 1966, at the age of twelve, Wayne beat out three hundred other students to win the prestigious Leverhulme Scholarship. Immediately after being awarded the honor, a required medical exam was scheduled where an X-ray of Wayne's ribs was to predict, within four inches, how tall he would eventually grow. Not having enough money to stay in London, Wayne and his family had to catch a train home to County Durham, forcing him to miss the medical appointment. By the time ballet officials realized the situation, it was too late to cancel the scholarship.

Dancing for over five decades, since the age of eight, Wayne often pushed his body beyond comfortable limits. The injuries that accompanied his dancing career were both inevitable and normal for a ballet dancer. Over the years, Wayne had torn cartilages and ligaments, a torn rotator cuff, fractured metatarsals, many groin strains, and Achilles tendon problems. Wayne considered getting used to the pain as part of the job.

Like many dancers, Wayne tried to ignore the warning signs from what he thought was a bad groin strain in 2003. A couple weeks of rest did not bring healing to his groin pain, nor his painful knee. Wayne continued to dance for several months in various plays and musicals. His passion and joy for dancing allowed him to cope with his pain. Wayne's excruciatingly painful knee, prompted him to get an X-ray. He was shocked to find out that his groin and knee pain were actually caused by his hip. Wayne learned that his hipbone was rubbing against his thighbone, because the cartilage that would normally cushion the two was completely deteriorated. Wayne's surgeon was mystified that he could continue to perform in Cabaret at the time. The desire to perform and not let his fans down enabled Wayne to keep going until he was limping, his back was aching, and he could barely walk, let alone dance in his next project, Cinderella. Wayne's right leg was in such bad shape that he could hardly raise it, and it was a struggle to get his shoes and socks on.

Finally reaching the point where performing was a nightmare, Wayne had to acknowledge that the constant pain had severely eroded his quality of life. Wayne's orthopedic surgeon recommended a hip replacement with a ceramic implant that came along with a ninety percent success rate. Wayne's surgeon chose a ceramic implant because it has a lower wear and failure rate in comparison to traditional metal and plastic implants. Knowing he was unable to endure the pain any longer, Wayne thought those odds sounded pretty good and accepted his surgeon's advice.

My experience with groin and knee pain was eerily similar to that of Wayne Sleep. I would venture to guess that our two X-rays were close to identical, as was our passionate desire to continue dancing as long as possible, on severely painful, deteriorated hips.

Had I known about Wayne's experience with pain, and his chronology of revelations that led to his hip replacement surgery, I would not have wasted thousands of my dollars chasing false hopes and believing in frivolous miracle cures. I would not have wasted a year on a chiropractor who insisted that I did not have a hip problem. Nor would I have wasted numerous appointments with orthopedic doctors who encouraged me to do physical therapy, have strange solutions injected into my hip, and take drugs for a severely damaged hip with no cartilage.

Certainly, Wayne Sleep and Darla Davies are not the only individuals to ever present symptoms of severe groin pain, soon after accompanied by intense knee pain. These symptoms must have been seen in hundreds of thousands of patients who frequently visit chiropractors, Rolfers, physical therapists, and orthopedic doctors throughout the United States and Europe. Why is this information not universal amongst these specialists? It seems like such a simple, basic, equation: $x + y = z$. Groin pain + knee pain = a hip problem! Duh.

Chronic groin pain alone should be a huge hint to any intelligent, observant individual that there is a hip problem. Apparently, this is not common knowledge among all doctors and therapists, so hear it from me now. I want to help you to avoid the painful, expensive journey that I limped through for so many months. If you have unrelenting chronic groin pain, followed by developing knee pain, then you should suspect a hip problem and get the hip X-rayed. Also know that there are currently no miracle cures or injections that are going to magically fix a severely damaged and worn out hip joint that has no cartilage.

In addition to his hip problem, Wayne Sleep also struggled with a moral dilemma. After twenty years he was honored to accept an invitation to perform as a guest at the Royal Opera House, dancing the role of the ugly sister, in the ballet *Cinderella*. Wayne's hip replacement surgery was scheduled for January, which would give him only three months to recover. Having made the commitment, a year prior,

Wayne was uncertain as to whether he should reveal his plans for hip replacement surgery to the ballet directors. He hoped and believed that he would be able to dance after the operation, but there were no guarantees. The question lingered: Would Wayne's new hip allow him to do the Charleston, in stiletto heels, with its characteristic high kicks, such a short time after hip replacement surgery? Or would he end up in a wheelchair, with one leg shorter than the other, and walk with a permanent limp? Wayne knew that the situation was beyond his control. All he could do was surrender himself to the surgeon and hope.

Wayne's hip replacement surgery was on January 7, which is my birthday. How weird is that? Having become so accustomed to chronic pain, Wayne was thrilled to find that it was eliminated after the operation, even after the pain medication had worn off. Up on crutches the day after surgery, Wayne felt as though his back, groin, and knee pain had miraculously disappeared. After five days, Wayne left the hospital with a stern warning to follow the "hip rules," which would determine the outcome of his new hip. Wayne followed the rules religiously in spite of the frustration and consequences. Wayne was not allowed to bend his knees or squat. When sitting, he was cautioned not to let the knees rise above a ninety-degree angle for fear that the hip would dislocate and the operation would have to be redone. When lying down, Wayne had to put a pillow between his legs to stop him from bending or crossing his legs, which could dislocate the hip as well. Six weeks of little movement more than a bit of walking caused Wayne to pile on the weight. In addition, he lost the strength in his thighs as all of the muscles had atrophied.

Wayne felt a sense of urgency as time was running out and *Cinderella* was only a few weeks away. Wayne attacked his new fitness regime with full force. He swam twenty-four laps a day. Unable to do breaststroke because it required bending the legs and caused added strain on the hip, Wayne did breaststroke, with his arms only, while paddling his legs up and down. Wayne spent hours at the gym, working with weights, and doing Pilates to strengthen his core muscles. His strong discipline enabled Wayne to lose all of the extra weight.

The skeptical ballet directors had been observing Wayne's progress during the last three weeks of his rehabilitation. There was a question as to whether he would regain the strength and fitness to open the show. One final medical exam would be the deciding factor in determining whether his contract for *Cinderella* could be ratified. After three months of therapy and rehabilitation, Wayne's surgeon was hesitant to confirm that Wayne would even be capable of the required material, along with the hours of rehearsals. Wayne was so fearful and nervous about doing his first jump. In practice, Wayne and the other "ugly sister" linked arms, and tentatively jumped two full circles of fifty contiguous jumps. These jumps in high heels were extremely difficult for Wayne, and he was deeply concerned about the banging on the hip joint. Wayne felt so good to be dancing again, and the onlookers were even more elated.

Wayne continued with aggressive sessions of physical therapy, punishing hours of exercise, and full rehearsals. At age sixty-two, three months after hip replacement surgery, he was back on stage at the Royal Opera House, dancing the role of an Ugly Sister in the ballet of *Cinderella*. Wayne referred to himself as Britain's bionic dancer. Having been in pain for the past seven years, he was finally pain free and felt as though he was walking on air. Wayne had known that it was such a high risk to have hip replacement surgery so close to his Royal Ballet comeback. He was fearful that he might not be able to walk again, let alone produce high-level quality dancing. A skilled surgeon and diligent pursuit of therapy and training seemed to be the key for Wayne Sleep's success.

Wayne Sleep's impressive comeback was a huge boost to my confidence and belief in the possibility of my own future comeback. My biggest task was going to be to propel myself forward and backward across the dance floor, in two-and-a-half inch heels, along with a few developés and rondés, with one leg or the other.

I said to myself, "If this guy can do fifty contiguous leaps in stiletto heels only three months after his hip replacement surgery, then I can certainly be back on the ballroom dance competition floor, in winning form, seven months after my hip replacement surgery! Thank you, Wayne. I believe!"

## Chapter 11

# Time to Get Serious

The real glory is being knocked to your knees and then
coming back. That's the real glory.

**—Vince Lombardi**

It was about five weeks after my surgery that I decided it was time to graduate to more demanding rehabilitation. My intention was to be back on the competition floor within the next six or seven months. I knew that getting my strength back was going to take some hard work, so it was time for me to get serious and motivated.

I knew of a few ballroom dancers who had returned to teaching and competing with their new hips. Although I could see that they were getting along fairly well, I did not see them out there consistently, nor were they moving with the strength and the power that is required by top level dancers.

I did have some lingering doubts that crept into my head once in a while. Could I, with a hip replacement at my age, come back to compete and win against the best Pro Am dancing couples in the country?

Dr. Wise's cutting words continued to haunt me: "You will be able to walk, but you will not dance again."

Although Dr. Wise annoyed me with his lack of encouragement and poor bedside manner, I almost have to thank him for lighting a fighting fire inside of me. I wanted to prove Dr. Wise wrong, and show him that great things are possible for hip replacement recipients. I did not need any negative, ignorant people dragging me down. I wanted to choose my mentors and cheerleaders wisely, and surround myself with only positive influences. My focus was on moving forward with my goal to get back to the competition floor, and ultimately win another United States Championship title.

Golfer, Tom Watson was the only over fifty athlete that I knew of who had come back with a new hip to compete at the top of his game against the best in his sport. Watson, at age fifty-nine, with his new hip, came so close to winning the 2009 British Open. Impressive, yes, however, Tom did not have to haul his butt backwards down the dance floor in high heels! As I pondered about what it would take for me to be at the top of my game, I knew that I would need to produce a lot more movement than merely walking or shuffling around a casual social dance floor. I needed to create the leg strength to move with speed and power on this new hip. That is what it would take for me to win.

I decided that I should have a motivational phrase or motto to say to myself when I was feeling fearful or doubtful. An aficionado of butterflies since I was a young girl, I likened my situation to an injured butterfly wanting to fly again.

I thought, *the butterfly with the broken wing will fly twice as high.* That's it! That phrase would become my comfort, my strength, and my mantra.

I was having dinner with a friend one evening, and she asked me, "Do you really think that you are going to come back from this surgery and beat all of those strong ladies who are out there winning now?"

Feeling slightly annoyed by her question, I remained polite, as I straightened out my friend.

"Sure, why not? My hip will be solid, strong titanium. I will have the power to move like never before."

My friend's silence told me that she really was not part of my A Team. I smiled as I looked her straight in the eyes, and said, "The butterfly with the broken wing will fly twice as high."

My friend just smirked and changed the direction of our dinner conversation. I was assembling an A Team of believers, and a B Team of non-believers. This friend was just demoted to the B Team, along with Dr. Wise. They could wallow together in their tub of negativity, while I traveled with my A Team onward, toward the path to victory.

My home physical therapist encouraged me to move on to a more specialized therapy program, and recommended an orthopedic rehabilitation specialist. My new therapist, Chris, had played on the same tennis team with me a few years prior, so she was surprised to see me show up one day as her new patient. Chris was both enthusiastic and positive. She had no doubts that I would be dancing again within a few months.

I was still walking with a cane, and feeling sore and unbalanced, so Chris started me out with some very basic exercises designed to help me establish basic body control and stability. Lying down, I would do side leg lifts with ankle weights. Lying on my back with a big rubber band wrapped around my thighs, I did "bridges" by raising my butt off the floor and lowering it back down. As my leg strength slowly returned, I was able to do semi-squat side steps, back and forth across the room.

Hip rehab is not merely about regaining leg strength. Strengthening the trunk muscles of the body is equally important. This is a key area of focus for dancers who are always talking about working and using the "core" of their bodies to produce movement.

Doing exercises while standing on a BOSU® ball was an interesting challenge. The BOSU® is half of a big exercise ball that has a flat hard surface on one side. I would attach a big rubber band to the exercise bar while standing on the round part of the ball. I slowly pulled each end of the band back toward my hips, and then slowly released them, while maintaining the tension with the band. I also did this standing sideways, pulling the two ends of the band in one hand across my body. Easier said than done.

The swimming pool was a fun alternative to the gym routine. Merely walking forward, backward, and sideways was beneficial. I did hip circles and figure eight motions with each leg. Other leg exercises included hamstring curls, heel and toe raises, straight leg raises, leg swings to the side, bicycle movements, and flutter kicks.

I also did a series of arm exercises in the pool using plastic hand weights. One can get a really good workout by holding the weights under the water and swinging the arms in various patterns.

Nearly two months after my surgery, I felt as though I was making steady progress, however I knew that if I wanted to be competing in another five months, I would need to kick it all up a notch. Unlike Dr. Wise, Chris seemed so confident that I would soon be dancing again on my new hip. There were times when I felt that she believed in me more than I believed in myself. I continued to mumble my phrase of comfort to myself many times throughout each day. *The butterfly with the broken wing will fly twice as high.* I had to keep encouraging myself, because I still had pain, and my balance was really off at times.

I never thought that two months after hip replacement surgery, I would be jogging in place on a BOSU® ball. I also did pendulum leg swings, mini sits, and overhead lifts with a light bar while standing on the BOSU® ball. Chris encouraged me to push myself, without losing recognition and respect for the hip precautions.

I really felt like I was making some significant progress when I was able to do a series of exercises on the six-inch riser platform. I started with basic side dips, while standing with one leg on the platform. I used a long wooden stick, called a dowel for balance, like one would use a cane. I never imagined that at this point in my recovery, I would be jumping up and down off of this thing. Although I completely trusted Chris, there were times when she would instruct me to do something, and I would look at her smiling and ask, "Are you serious?"

Chris would return the smile, and assuredly respond, "Of course."

I was able to do a series of exercise patterns, like quick steps forward and back, off of the riser, stepping up and over the top, to the other side, and also straddling the riser, stepping up with one leg after the other, and down again. I was amazed that I was doing several sets of ten, for each of these exercises.

On the big exercise ball, I was given an array of leg and arm exercises, some of which involved sitting on the ball and using hand weights. Also included were some leg lifts while lying on my stomach on top of the ball, and some leg lifts, lying backward with just my shoulders supported on the ball.

I was beginning to feel so elated with my command of my rehab exercise program. I was feeling confident and positive until I was presented with the elusive "bird dog" exercise. This particular task made me feel frustrated and depressed. This one, stupid exercise made me question whether I really would be able to dance on this new hip. *Maybe Dr. Wise was right. Maybe I would not be able to dance again. No, No, No! The butterfly with the broken wing will fly twice as high!*

The "bird dog" exercise seemed so simple, yet required some leg strength and balance. Standing on one leg and pointing the other leg backward, one bends forward reaching and stretching forward the same arm as the standing leg, while holding a small ball. I could do this quite well on my non-surgical, right leg, however, trying to accomplish this while standing on my left leg, was almost a comedy routine. I would attempt this feat four to five times a week at the gym. Month after month, I could not do it, even once, without losing my balance and falling over. My left leg was still so weak. I worked in a small corner of the gym, unnoticed I thought, yet still found myself looking around in embarrassment, to see who might be watching my ridiculous show. I felt so uncoordinated, and on the verge of crying sometimes. Certainly, my therapist would not have given me an exercise that was unreasonable or unattainable. I kept trying to do the "bird dog" over and over again, week after week. Finally, after four, frustrating months I mastered the pose, holding the ball proudly in front of myself, without falling over. A small victory for this hip replacement patient, yet a giant step in my mind. I often wondered how other athletes made it through this process, because it was not easy.

 **DARLA'S TIPS FOR**

## Rehabilitation

1. Take action in your healing and set realistic goals.
2. Remember, slow and steady wins the race. Use a rational and systematic rehabilitation program. This will lesson your chances of injury to your new hip, and enable you to eventually return to your sport with strength and confidence.
3. Exercise every day and keep a positive attitude.

## Chapter 12

# Back in the Ball Gown Again

Life isn't about waiting for the storm to be over,
it's about learning how to dance in the rain.
**—Author Unknown**

About four months after my surgery, I progressed to basic dance steps and drills along with my gym exercises. Jim and I took it slowly by just doing the basic Waltz and Foxtrot for a couple of weeks. I was naturally fearful about placing my full weight on my left leg with that new hip. It felt odd and somewhat weak at first, but when I realized that I was not going to fall over, I became more confident.

I was anxious to try some Cha Cha and Rumba to test my Cuban hip action. Prior to my hip surgery, that hip rotation in the Rhythm dances was really painful.

One day I stood in front of the mirror at the dance studio and thought, *This is it; this will be the true test of my new hip: a nice, slow, Rumba box step.* I recalled the piercing pain that I had experienced the last time that I had tried to make my hips do those Rumba boxes. Trying to forget the past, I took a step back on my right leg, settled my weight, and pulled my right hip back. Next, I stepped sideways on my left leg. I was so afraid. I wondered if my new left hip was going to accept the weight and the required hip rotation. My excitement was building as I settled my weight onto my left leg and pulled my left hip back. As I closed my right foot to my left, settled my weight, and pulled my right hip back, I looked in the mirror feeling absolutely delighted as I saw my own smile looking back at me.

A couple of private dance lessons were underway in the studio while I was in the corner making this earthshaking discovery. Unable to contain my excitement, I turned around and shouted at anyone who would listen, "It doesn't hurt anymore! No more pain! I can do a Rumba box and it doesn't hurt!"

They all chuckled, and shared in my extreme elation. Just to be sure, I did Rumba boxes, and Cucarachas for another ten minutes. My reflection in the mirror was still smiling back at me.

After dancing moderately in my very low-heeled practice shoes for about a month-and-a-half, I switched over to my two-and-a-half-inch high heels. The transition was not a problem, and I was feeling sturdy and confident. Soon Jim and I went back to practicing our Waltz, Tango, Foxtrot, and Viennese Waltz routines.

Although my left leg was so much stronger than what it had been prior to the surgery, there was lingering muscular pain. During hip replacement surgery, the muscles around the hip are cut, and it can take over a year for them to reattach and mold around the titanium implant. I could live with this small amount of muscular pain, because it was nothing compared to the debilitating joint pain that I had endured in the past.

Seven months after my surgery, Dr. Hedley assured me that my X-ray looked perfect, and that any pain in my hip area was residual from what I had been dealing with prior to surgery. Dr. Hedley proudly encouraged me to go ahead and dance in competitions.

"Do anything you want. Just don't get tackled or slide into base," he said. We both laughed. No, I did not aspire to play football or baseball. I just wanted to be a competitive amateur ballroom dancer.

I was amazed at how well I was progressing with my new hip. Having been consistent with my physical therapy exercises, I was feeling both confident and capable. In spite of continued minor muscular soreness in the hip area, I was feeling reasonably well supported. I had been practicing my four smooth dance routines (Waltz, Tango, Foxtrot, and Viennese Waltz) for a few weeks, so it felt like the right time to try out my new hip at a competition. One might have expected me to feel apprehension and fear about dancing on the new hip after nearly a year off, but I was remarkably relaxed. Previous thoughts of tension and insecurity were replaced with uplifted feelings of strength and confidence—almost jubilation. I went from pain, weakness, and suffering to having it all erased. Certainly this must be qualified as a miracle. I felt like a jockey, who after a long recovery from an injury, was back in the saddle again and ready to ride the race. My leg was strong, and for the most part, pain free, and because of this, I could physically do more so my dancing was much improved. I looked forward to showing everyone how I could run down the dance floor like a fast horse (well, at least that is how I perceived it in my own mind).

I chose the Chicago Crystal Ball Competition for the debut of my new hip. I felt comfortable with this medium-sized competition for my first comeback attempt. Stamina is always a concern when one has to dance several one minute, fifteen second heats in a row. I would have to dance four heats with only a couple minutes to rest before dancing another four heats. This was not an ideal situation, because it had been eleven months since I had danced in a competition. I would much rather have danced the first four heats, and then had at least a fifteen or twenty minute rest before having to put out the energy to do it all again.

My hip and I handled the situation well, and I won all events that I entered, including the big multi-dance scholarship event so coveted by all Pro Am competitors.

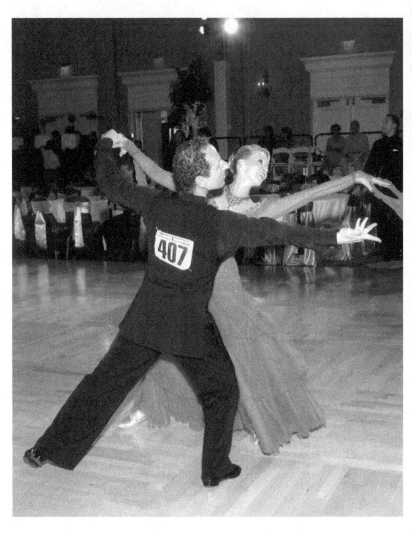

The Chicago Crystal Ball was my first competition with my new hip.
Seven months after my hip replacement surgery, I was relaxed and happy
as I placed first in all of my events.

For any doubters not believing that a hip replacement recipient can return to ballroom dancing at the top open gold level of Pro Am competition and win—believe it.

And to Dr. Wise who told me that I would never dance again, I wanted to say, "Hey, look at me now, Doc!"

I knew that from that day on the strength and quality of my dancing would continue to grow and improve, along with my leg strength. In the past, the evolvement of my technical dancing skills was thwarted by my chronic pain and physical limitations.

One of my coaches just happened to be on the judging panel at the Chicago competition. Afterward, she mentioned to Jim that although I did a great job for my first time with the new hip, it was important for me to show more independence in my dancing. Although it is true that the woman must wait for the man to lead her in ballroom dancing, much of the time she is dancing independently of him, and he catches up to her and sort of picks her up before they resume dancing as a couple. In the evolvement of my dancing education, it was essential for me to be able to hold myself up and maintain my own space while staying on time to the music, and still showing cohesiveness with my partner. It was time to grow up as a dancer. I could not always look to get back to my partner and grab him. Ha! I had to learn to be more aloof, and let him chase after me. From that day onward, I was going to be able to pedal the bike on my own, instead of just sitting there and coasting.

Our next competition was one of the largest, The Millennium DanceSport Championships in St. Petersburg, Florida. I felt pretty strong, although I still had lingering muscular soreness in my hip area. There were certain dance steps that caused me some discomfort. It was not excruciating pain; I was just made aware that this area around my new hip implant was not yet one hundred percent healed. When I did the step called the Standing Spin, I could feel it in my hip area as I pushed my feet in small steps around Jim. Another step called the Rondé caused discomfort as well. I kicked with my right leg, but my left leg felt the pressure as it supported my body weight. I hoped that as I continued to train at the gym, I would become stronger each week and eventually work through this issue. At times, I suppose I got a bit tentative with certain steps, which was not pleasing to Jim.

I wish I had a dollar for every time he said to me, "You are stumbling. You are not on your feet!"

Of course, I was not that bad. Jim just likes to use drama for shock value. Jim knew that I had a big goal and mediocrity was simply not good enough. I had to strive to be better than myself.

I placed second in my big scholarship event at that competition. This was a huge victory for me, as I stood behind the undefeated champion. Nobody had been able to dethrone this queen in this division, so I was thrilled with my great result.

Our next competition was the International Grand Ball in San Francisco, California. My increasing strength and confidence helped me to win all of my events easily.

The Midwest was our next destination for the Heart of America Championships. In spite of a good, strong performance, I placed fifth in my big scholarship event. There was no obvious reason for this disappointing result. Clearly, I was not politically favored at that competition. Although the judges' scores are available for viewing, dancers are not permitted to approach judges and question their marks. One judge, who was not judging my event, just happened to be in the ballroom watching. Judging panels rotate every couple of hours, so she was just waiting to take her place on the next judging panel. This judge had judged me many times over the past few years. Having never received coaching from this judge, I was surprised when she went out of her way to come over to me and tell me how much she enjoyed my dancing. She confided that I was a fairly good dancer before, but admitted that she was shocked at my strong improvement.

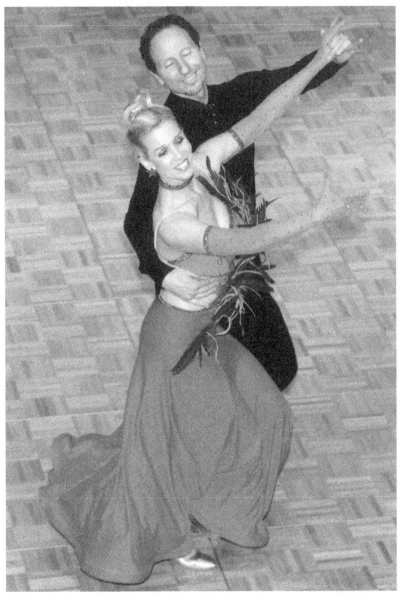

My return to the U.S. Dance Championships eleven months after hip replacement surgery proved that I was a top contender. I was not displeased with my fifth place finish; however, I continued to believe that I would win again.

Perplexed, she asked, "Wow! What happened?"

I was so flattered, and her comments made me feel so much better after my undesired fifth-place finish. I explained to her that I had had a hip replacement ten months prior, and it felt like I had a whole new leg. My newfound leg strength was obvious to me, but what a delight that others could recognize this transformation in my dancing. This was all that I needed to fuel my competitive spirit and move onward.

The Nevada Star Ball was our next stop on the competition circuit. I had come a long way in ten short months, and I was feeling positive and powerful. Once again, I placed first in my big event. This result was especially satisfying, as I beat one of the reigning queens in the American Smooth division. There were about five or six women who had politically staked claims on the placements in this division over the past couple of years. Having been missing in action for nearly eleven months, I was happy to show that I was not only back, but also back to win.

Ten months and one week after my hip replacement surgery, I was competing at the United States DanceSport Championships. All of the top dancers were present, and each one of us had the ability and the potential to be the winner. After three rounds of dancing, the final seven couples chosen were called back to the floor to dance the deciding round. Sometimes, even the best dancers get shut out of a big final, so I was thrilled when our number was called. All of the women finalists had blond hair, so people were referring to this showdown as the "battle of the blonds." I knew that I was up against a very tough lot, but I really felt as though I had danced my personal best. I was not disappointed with my fifth place finish, yet on the other hand, it was not what I wanted. I wanted to win. I knew that it was a very good accomplishment for me to come back and make it into that final less than a year after hip replacement surgery. I gave myself a pep talk telling myself that it was just going to take another year. I would have to put those proverbial overalls on again and get back to work

It is hard to keep yourself from getting down when you feel as though you got ripped off and did not receive your just rewards. Nobody wins all the time—not even the greatest athletes—so you have to learn to accept the bad results with the good ones. A disappointing result can be more difficult to deal with in dancing, because the reasons will likely never be known. Not only that, the reason for a failure could be due to political favor, and have nothing whatsoever to do with one's dancing performance. In other sports, the contestants either get the ball in or over, and produce the best score, or win the event by moving the fastest or jumping the highest. The winner in many sports is decided by specific actions, whereas in ballroom dancing, the winner is determined merely by the judges opinions, preferences, likes, and dislikes, which can be based on practically anything.

I have seen many dancers pout, give up, and quit dancing when they did not make a certain achievement within a limited time period. Too many dancers either think that they are deserving of the accolades without doing the work, or are just too lazy to do the work that is required to make it to the top. Some are so close, yet are not willing to do all of the little detailed things that it takes to make them a winner.

When I am feeling low or discouraged, I like to read the following poem by an unknown author, which I always keep in my handbag.

## DON'T QUIT

When things go wrong, as they often will
When the road you're trudging seems all uphill
When the funds are low and the debts are high
When you want to smile but you have to sigh
When care is pressing you down a bit
Rest if you must but don't you quit

Life is queer with its twists and turns
As every one of us sometimes learns

And many a fellow turns about
When he might have won had he stuck it out
Don't give up though the pace seems slow
You may succeed with another blow
Often the goal is nearer than
It seems to a faint and faltering man
Often the struggler has given up
When he might have captured the victor's cup
And he learned too late when the night came down
How close he was to the golden crown
Success is failure turned inside out
The silver tint of the clouds of doubt
And you never can tell how close you are
It may be near when it seems so far
So stick to the fight when you're hardest hit
It's when things seem worse that you must not quit
For all the sad words of tongue or pen
The saddest are these: "It might have been!"

I always feel inspired and rejuvenated after reading this poem. Often I will leave copies of it lying around the dance studio in hopes that it will fall into the hands of someone who really needs to hear it. Whoever wrote this poem should feel such satisfaction for having touched the hearts and revived the spirits of all who have embraced it.

Sometimes, all it takes is hearing a simple phrase from a favorite mentor. I never forgot this one statement that Oprah Winfrey made in a television interview. She said, "I always believed that I was born for greatness."

I remember feeling so in awe of her confidence and unyielding belief in herself and her abilities. I considered Oprah a member of my A Team.

Like Oprah, I chose to believe big. I believed that I would have future dancing moments of greatness.

## DARLA'S TIPS FOR

### Getting Back into Your Sport

1. Do not allow challenges and difficulties to cause you to become discouraged or to give up on your dreams.
2. Keep your passion and your enthusiasm.
3. Believe that another victory is coming your way.

## Chapter 13

# Kicking It All Up a Notch

> Don't let what you cannot do
> interfere with what you can do.
> **—John Wooden**

Having completed my first competition with my new hip, I was feeling excited about my dancing future. I thought to myself, *if I was able to dance that well only seven months after surgery, and my hip was not even one hundred percent healed, then how much improved could my dancing be after I added some serious strength training to my daily workouts?*

I chose my personal trainer, Derek, because he has a degree in sports medicine with an emphasis on biomechanics. Most importantly, as a certified physical therapist, Derek is aware of the precautions and limitations required for athletes who have had joint replacements.

I showed Derek my basic dance position, and explained to him how a dancer must hold her "dance frame," with arms held wide, and body lifted, with an arch in the upper back. This is not an easy task for lady dancers, as we all have a tendency to let the left arm drop, or allow a shoulder to cave inward, or allow the body to rotate too much. Equally as important as a strong, uplifted dance frame, is for a dancer to show leg strength and power while moving across the floor. Improving my overall strength was going to improve the quality of my dancing.

I told Derek that he was going to train me to be the first hip replacement recipient to win a United States Ballroom Dance Championship, and perhaps the first hip replacement recipient to win a national championship in any traveling movement sport. Derek loved the idea! He was definitely onboard to be on my A Team of cheerleaders. It was going to be a fun project, probably more so for Derek than for me. I had witnessed the torture that was in store for me.

For years, I had watched Derek train other athletes at the gym while I kept to my safe non-strenuous workouts. I was intimidated, thinking that surely I was not strong enough to do most of those things, especially not with a new hip! A tennis player friend of mine had been working out with Derek for a year. Loving the experience and her results, she encouraged me to get a program going with Derek. I did not want to seem like a wimp, and I really wanted to add a new dimension to my dancing. Although I secretly dreaded it, I knew that I must follow this path in order to gain strength and power. Derek was one of those characters who was going to help me travel down the "yellow brick road" and find my way to Oz.

Derek designed and developed workout plans for me, which focused on four important areas: agility, core strength, upper body strength, and leg strength. There were times when Derek would set up a task for me to do, and I would look at him in disbelief and say, "You are kidding, right?" Or I would ask him, "Are you sure I'm allowed to do that with my hip?" Or feeling completely over faced, I would say, "I really don't think I will be able to do that."

Derek would just smile and say, "You can, and you will."

Honestly, I found myself shocked after accomplishing some tasks that I never would have imagined possible for me and my new hip. Yet,

I must say, it was not all pleasant. There were times when I wanted to give up, as I lay down on the floor protesting.

"I can't. I won't. Please don't torture me like this!"

Derek would say to me, "Do you want to win? Or would you rather place fifth or sixth?"

End of discussion. That is all Derek had to say to stop my complaining. I wanted to win at every competition. Making it to the final round of six winners is an accomplishment that any top dancer should be proud of, however, having studied sports psychology in the past, I had a winning mindset. I wanted to place first, not second, third, or fourth, and certainly not fifth or sixth.

My workouts typically began with an eight-to-ten minute warm up on one of the cardio machines. The elliptical machine is a fusion of a stair climber and cross-country ski machine. As one stands on it and pedals, it mimics the motion of running without the impact on the legs and feet.

The rowing machine might look easy because one is sitting, but trust me, it requires high energy, and forces one to really use both the arms and legs.

The step mill was the most challenging of the cardio machines for me. Unlike the elliptical, where one can get away with slacking off and reducing one's effort, the step mill's revolving staircase forces one to keep moving. I was afraid of the step mill because it required more of an effort for me to lift my left leg, which still had a tendency to be weak and lazy. Derek insisted that I not use the side rail for support, and swing my arms freely as though I were walking. I was terrified. My fear of tripping and possibly falling forced me to dig up some extra energy and concentration.

Derek always put the resistance setting on these machines much higher than I would have chosen for myself. It was tough, and sometimes I wondered if I could get through just five minutes much less ten of this initial warm-up exercise. I was always glad when the warm up was over, but often wondered how I would make it through the next hour and fifteen minutes of our training session. I tried to tantalize myself with visual images of me standing on the podium at a big competition, with a big trophy in my hand. It also helped me to look forward to a trip to Starbucks as a reward after these demanding workouts.

Derek gave me some mobilization exercises that went beyond the basic stretching and squatting tasks that I was given during my early rehabilitation. Déjà vu. There I was again, in the middle of the gym, losing my balance and falling over in the midst of scrutinizing strangers. The purpose of the Frankenstein walk was to mobilize the hips and hamstrings. Standing with one arm extended horizontally in front of my body, I had to slowly kick my opposite leg (keeping it straight) up to touch my hand. Easier said than done, and certainly not pain free for me. Merely maintaining my balance for this task was a challenge. Trying to keep these walks going back and forth across the gym a couple of times, turned me into a frustrated Frankenstein.

The lunge targets mobilization of the hips and thighs. Like the Frankenstein walks, this exercise requires balance and coordination. I took a stride forward on to a flat foot, while keeping my body upright with shoulders back. Bending both legs I dropped my rear knee close to the floor, and then pushed myself up with my front heel to standing position. Again, it is not as easy as it looks like it should be, and it is uncomfortable and challenging to one who has weak legs and a new hip. A couple of times across the gym had me wanting to scream, "No more!"

As the weeks passed, my legs were gaining some strength and my balance was improving. One day, Derek decided to add squat jumps to my program.

"You really are joking this time, right?" I really thought he was pulling my leg. Walking the lunges was bad enough, and now I was expected to do leaping lunges across the gym! The rolling of Derek's eyes told me that he was really serious. I sensed that Derek was annoyed and disappointed in me for acting like a wimp and not trusting him. I tried to toughen up as I pressed onward.

In the area of agility or functional training, I did several exercises on the step platforms. The lateral hurdle step and the lateral box step over were very challenging, especially when I was jumping up and down off the platform with my left leg leading. Stepping forward up and back down quickly from the platform many times is exhausting. Nearly stumbling a few times was alarming. Even more frightening was approaching the platform laterally from a side step, traveling the length of three feet across the platform, to touch the floor with my foot on the other side, and then quickly back again to the other side. After completing a set of twenty and feeling exhausted, I was just relieved to have made it through that one. When Derek told me I had to do three more sets of twenty, I just looked at him in disbelief. *That's eighty total reps. There's no way!* I thought. *I had a hip replacement how many months ago? I am how old?*

I was being treated like some jock athlete in the middle of a rigorous training program. It felt so surreal to me that I was actually doing, what I was doing, after total hip replacement surgery. It seemed amazing that what I was experiencing at that moment was even possible. Somehow, I made it through forty repetitions on each leg without falling or calling 9-1-1.

There were a couple of exercises that I actually enjoyed because they were less painful and more closely related to dancing movement. The speed ladder, an actual ladder that lies on the ground, is an excellent dance-training tool. I had fun doing the "carioca" step in and out of the rungs of the long ladder, back and forth across the aerobics room several times. This is similar to the "grapevine" step that we do in the Foxtrot. Traveling sideways to the left for example, I crossed my right leg in front of my left leg, and then took a side step with my left, followed by crossing my right leg behind the left leg. Each step crossed over the rungs of the ladder. I had to take big, strong, steps, with accuracy to avoid stumbling or falling down.

Another exercise I did on the speed ladder reminded me of the childhood game of hopscotch. Starting at one end of the ladder, I jumped with both feet into the middle of one square, and then jumped forward again splitting my legs, landing my feet outside the next square. Six times across the aerobics room is a lot of jumping. This is not an exercise you will want to do if you have just had a lot of coffee or water to drink.

The Reebok slide was another fun exercise for balance and agility. Designed to mimic the movement of Olympic speed skaters, this low impact exercise tones the inner and outer thighs, as well as the gluteal muscles. A wonderful tool for a hip replacement patient, this exercise strengthens the ligaments of the hip and knee joints, thus improves hip stability and balance. I put these special booties on over my shoes and glided from side to side, with big powerful sweeping strides, on a long, flat slide board. Having ice-skated a fair amount in my past, I was able to adapt quickly to the balance and movement required for this task.

At first glance, one might have thought that Derek was training a basketball player, as we ran through the lateral lane slide. This is a great agility exercise for dancers as well, because it requires transferring body weight and changing direction quickly. Working on a straight line, Derek would roll a small ball several feet to my right. I had to crouch down, keeping my butt low, with a straight back and my head up. I took shuffle steps (similar to dance chases) over to the ball, scooped it up, and pitched it back to Derek. Immediately, I had to shuffle step quickly back over to the left side to grab the ball and continue on with the exercise.

Core strength is very important for ballroom dancers. A strong center is necessary to raise the upper body from the waist up, and sink the lower body into the ground from the waist down. I never looked forward to the painful abdominal exercises. I did the back extension exercise on the physio ball. Lying with abs and thighs across the ball, and legs extended with toes touching the floor, and tips of the fingers touching the sides of my head, I slowly straightened and raised my upper body, then gently lowered it to the starting position.

I also did this back extension exercise on the Roman chair, which is an apparatus that has a ledge at the base where you can secure your feet. I was positioned facedown on the apparatus, with the back of my calves hooked under the rollers, and the tops of my thighs on the front pads. With my hands behind my neck, I lowered my torso to the floor, while keeping my back straight. Then I used my butt muscles to slowly raise my body upward. I did side bends on the Roman chair as well. Lying sideways on the apparatus, with my feet secured on the ledge, and hands held at head level, I leaned slowly sideways toward the floor, and then raised my body back up to the start position.

The medicine ball side throw was another fun exercise, although not a piece of cake. Standing on a line, with Derek positioned several feet behind me, and diagonal to my right shoulder, I pivoted left, rotating my body around to face Derek with my arms extended straight in front of my body. Catching a medicine ball thrown by Derek, I pivoted to the right, while holding the ball up and extended, all the way around to face Derek, then again rotated back around to the left (maintaining the ball on an even plane), releasing the ball with power back to Derek.

Once again, it seemed like it should be an easy exercise, but the weight of the ball made it tough to maintain body control. I was required to release the ball with straight arms; bending the arms and throwing the ball was not acceptable for Derek. *He's so demanding. So particular!* I thought. If I messed up and lost my balance, or dropped the ball before I completed ten repetitions, Derek would make me start all over with number one. I got so frustrated, because sometimes I was close to the finish and fell over on the eighth or ninth rep, which meant that I to start all over again. Consequently, sometimes I would have to do thirty or forty of these throws just to get ten in a row that were acceptable.

I dreaded the Double V sit-ups. It was both difficult and painful to raise my body up to have my straight arm meet the opposite straight leg. It felt nearly impossible to keep going for more than a few repetitions, but somehow I struggled through the misery of this exercise.

The physio ball opposite superman's was another exercise that made me feel like a fool, as it presented the same balance issue for me as that crazy bird dog exercise from my early stages of rehabilitation. This one seemed like it should be easier as I was lying on my stomach on the big exercise ball. All I had to do was extend my opposite leg and arm, while maintaining balance with the fingertips and toes of the opposite limbs, in contact with the floor. It is funny how something that seems so basic and uncomplicated can be such a challenge and make one feel so uncoordinated.

Upper body strength is extremely important, as a dancer must maintain a strong, wide, uplifted dance frame. If a dancer's frame shows weakness or fatigue, it will cause loss of connection to her partner, thus the technique and quality of the dancing will suffer. The rowing machine is an excellent exercise for a dancer because it strengthens the upper back and builds stamina.

The upright row exercise also develops strength around the shoulder and upper back, and helps to improve posture. With feet hip-width apart, and a narrow overhand grip on the bar, I pulled the bar smoothly up toward my chin. I continued to pull the bar up with a straight back, to finish with my elbows high beside my head, and hands below my chin. After a brief pause, I lowered the bar to the start position with my arms fully extended.

The front side back exercise added strength and tone to my arms. Using five pound disc weights in each hand, I would extend them in front of my body to eye level, with straight arms parallel to the floor, and hold the pose a couple of seconds. Next I would raise both discs to eye level at either side of my body, and the final position was to extend the discs behind my back, while keeping my arms straight.

I am embarrassed to admit that I do not think I have ever been able to do a chin up. When Derek walked me over to the pull-up machine one day, I protested, telling him that I simply did not have the arm strength to do a pull-up. He explained that it was called the assisted pull-up machine, and on it, anyone can do pull-ups. The weight stack counters one's body weight, so I started out by lifting eighty percent of my body weight. *Oh, that's what it feels like to be strong, or at least look strong, and do a chin up.*

The bench press is not just for musclemen; dancers can do it too. Lying on a bench, I took an inverted grip on the weighted bar above my head. Pushing it up and keeping it stabilized was not easy. I had to slowly lower the bar to my chest, then quickly push it up, extending my arms straight. Derek actually had to help me lift the bar up the first couple of times. It was scary at first, but I really felt good after hoisting that thing up there on my own several times.

Derek added several exercises to my workout program to target the triceps muscles. Kneeling on a bench, supporting myself on my knee and arm, I did triceps kickbacks extending the opposite elbow behind my body. Slowly straightening my arm, I lifted a dumbbell to a horizontal position. After a brief pause, I slowly brought the dumbbell back down to start position. I could feel the burn after several sets of these.

I also did the triceps pushdown exercise. With knees slightly bent, feet flat and slightly apart, and my body held straight and upright, I reached for a bar at the end of a pulley. I had to push the bar down slowly, keeping my elbows close to my sides, pause at the bottom, and then slowly return to the start position. This is another one that looks like it should be so easy, but with added weights, it can be tough.

The plyometric step-up was another really tough exercise for me and my weak arms. Derek placed two large dumbbells with large side discs, on end, on the floor, shoulder width apart. I took a pushup position, with my hands flat on the floor, inside the dumbbells, and feet together. I placed one hand up on one dumbbell, followed by placing the other hand on the other dumbbell. I then brought one hand back down to the floor, followed by the other hand. I had to keep my core muscles tight and my back flat. My wrists were weak and my arms hurt. I hated this exercise, and told Derek I was afraid that I would break my little wrist. *Here it comes.* I cringed, as I knew Derek's lecture was coming.

"Darla, we can argue about it all you want, but you are going to do it." Ugh! That was a really tough one for me to get through.

I was excited to find out what kind of leg strength I could achieve with this new titanium hip. I knew that I would have to work at rebuilding the muscles in my hip area, and it would be a challenge, but anything would have to be an improvement over my painful past with my old hip. I attacked these leg exercises with sweat and tears, along with some light swearing at Derek here and there. Certainly nobody, including myself, would ever have imagined that a hip replacement patient would be using all of the leg machines typically seen in most gyms.

The seated leg press was a thrill for me because it looked so impossible for a hip replacement patient. As I sat on the machine, I was surprised that I had the leg strength to push the weighted plate away, extending my legs almost fully, before slowly returning to the start position. I could see the value of this exercise for building strength in the quads, hamstrings, and butt.

Sitting on the leg curl machine, I pulled the weight back with my ankles, contracting my hamstrings, and then returned it with control to the start position. On the leg extension machine, the weighted arm is on top of the ankles, instead of behind them, as on the curl machine. Thus the quad muscles were worked as I raised my lower legs to parallel the floor before returning to start position.

There were two hip machines at the gym that were extremely beneficial to me. They added strength to my butt and thighs, which my dancing would clearly show in the months to come. The hip abductor machine targets the muscles isolated on the outside of the thighs and buttocks. Seated, with my back supported, I pushed the weighted pads away from my body, with the outsides of my knees. Next, I would slowly resist the inward force, keeping the core of my body tight, as I slowly moved the pads back to the start position.

In my very early rehabilitation, I was not allowed to use the hip adductor machine, however after my new hip was healed, this machine became a valuable training tool. This exercise targeted the muscles of my inner thighs. Opposite to the hip abductor machine, I began with the weighted pads apart and used the inside of my knees and thighs to slowly push them together. Next, keeping my core muscles tense, I would return the pads to start position.

I was not fond of the bodyweight four corners exercise. It forced me to use my weak leg muscles, which was challenging and tough. I began by standing on my right leg, on a spongy, rubber, stability pad, with a big stick (dowel) in my right hand to use for balance. I had to bend into my right knee, pointing my straight left leg as far forward as possible. Next I had to point my left leg as far left as I could, while using the dowel to hold myself up. The third leg position was straight back, while getting way down in my right knee, and keeping my weight forward. The final position required me to twist as I brought my left leg behind my body and over to the right side, as far forward as possible. The real feat was doing this exercise while standing on my left leg, with my new hip. It was sort of painful, just because my leg muscles did not want to do this work. It was not that I absolutely could not do it, but more that I found it unpleasant, and just would rather not have to produce the effort.

I protested to Derek. "This is just too hard for me."

Keeping my goal in mind, Derek showed no mercy as he lectured me. "Darla, you can sit on your ass and hope and dream, but if you want to win, you must get up and do the work."

I sighed heavily. Of course Derek was right. I took a swig of water, grabbed the dowel, and proceeded onward with fricken bodyweight four corners.

The physio ball wall squats also required some extra work from my new left hip. I stood with the big ball behind my back, against the wall. My legs were positioned far enough in front of me so my lower legs were perpendicular to the ground when I squatted down and touched my fingertips to the floor. My left hip did not want to do this, but together, we got through it and got it done.

Derek had me doing things that I had seen big power lifters doing at the gym. Things that I never imagined I could be doing with a new hip. The high pull looked scary, but I thought it was pretty cool when I got the hang of it. Standing with my feet apart, I held the weighted bar, with my hands just outside my hips. I squatted down in a position like I was ready to dive into a pool, as I held the bar just above my knees. Next I jumped up, pulling the bar quickly up to my collarbone, and then I lowered the bar, as I concentrated on maintaining my upright stance.

The front squats to press was another exercise that made me feel like I was keeping up with the big boys. I stood upright holding the weighted bar against my thighs. From there I sat down on a stool behind me, then immediately stood, and thrust the bar over my head, with arms extended, while looking up. After holding the position for a couple of seconds, I lowered the bar to my chest. *Okay, I'm ready for the Olympics!* I thought.

The trap bar squats really made me feel like I was building muscles and getting strong. I stood inside this metal apparatus. I proceeded to squat down keeping my chest up, my back straight, and my feet flat. I grabbed the handles and lifted the bar as I stood up, extending my hip and knee to full extension. *A wimp, no more.*

Often, the day after these strenuous workouts, my leg muscles would be so very sore. This was actually a delight to me, because the soreness was not from the haunting joint pain of my past. This muscle soreness was building my strong legs of the future.

As the weeks passed, my increasing leg strength had a profound effect on not only the power element of my dancing, but the musical quality of my dancing. A non-dancer might not understand how a new hip, combined with newfound leg strength could improve my musical expression of a dance. How could leg strength, or the lack thereof, be related to musical timing? Being on time to the music that one is hearing is the most difficult thing to achieve in ballroom dancing. Many dancers disregard timing, by thinking that movement and power are more important. The wisest dance masters will tell you that being in sync with the music is different than marching to the beat. A dancing couple must show harmony of movement between each other, along with an expressive interpretation of the music.

In the past, my weak leg prevented me from maintaining my balance, while transferring my weight from one leg to the other. Consequently, I would lose my body control, thus arrive either too early, or too late, on a beat of music. One cannot listen to the music and demonstrate musical expressive dancing, if she cannot hold herself up and demonstrate controlled and balanced movement. In ballroom dancing, one's body movement does not stop with a step. The body actually continues the movement, until forced to take another step, which is dictated by the next beat of music. The average spectator of ballroom dancing would probably never imagine that things like core strength, upper body strength, and leg strength, and overall body control, have a direct impact on a dancer's ability to stay on time to the music, and fill it out as they say with musical expression.

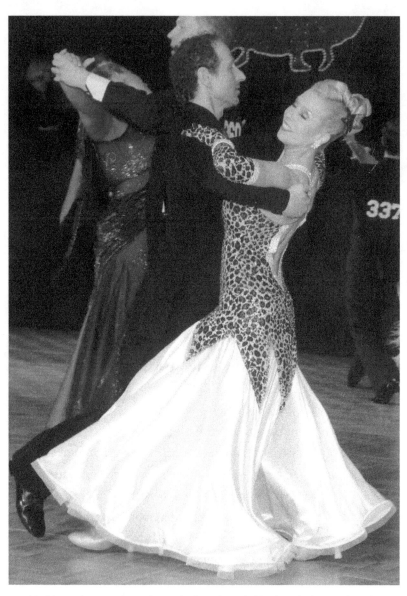

My hip replacement made me feel as though I had a whole new leg. As time passed, my increased leg strength improved the overall quality of my dancing.

The hip replacement did so much more for me than just take the debilitating pain away. It enabled me to create strength in my legs, which had not been possible prior to surgery. The newfound leg strength not only allowed me to execute my dance steps with more precision and power, but also allowed me to maintain my balance more consistently. Who would have guessed that a hip replacement would allow me to develop the tools necessary to add so many new dimensions to my dancing? For me, the hip replacement was proving to be so much more than something that was just fixed or patched up. It was like going from black and white to a world of many colors.

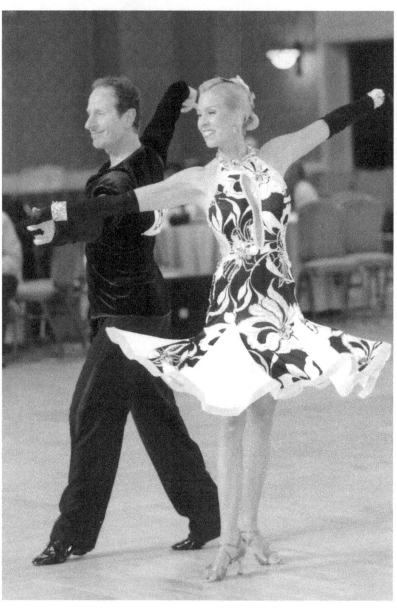

After competing in the American Smooth division for a year after my surgery, strength training gave me the confidence to return to the American Rhythm division as well.

**DARLA'S TIPS OF**

## Encouragement

1.  There will be days when you might feel like crying because everything seems painful and difficult. You must step away from discouragement and complacency, and strive for more than mediocrity. You must gather the strength to pick yourself up. I love this little ditty from Psalm 30 that my A Team member, Joel Osteen pointed out one day: *Weeping may endure for a night, but joy is coming in the morning.* Learn to press on and see yourself as strong and enduring.

2.  You must surround yourself with people who inspire you to rise higher. Your vision of who you want to become will be greatly impacted by the individuals you choose to associate with, so choose only those who support your dream.

## Chapter 14

# Age Is Just a Number

You are never too old to set another goal,
or to dream a new dream.

**—C.S. Lewis**

Overcoming hip replacement surgery to compete at the highest level, against the best in the country, was a lofty goal in itself. Was I crazy to believe that I could possibly go so far as to win a U.S. championship, with this new hip, at my age? I had to face the facts. I was not twenty, thirty, or even forty. I was over fifty! In spite of my age, which I chose not to see as a negative, I was feeling good, and I was becoming stronger and more skilled with each passing week. I felt in my heart that I should keep pressing onward with my goal.

Advances in medicine and science have enabled many athletes to extend their athletic careers. Orthopedic medicine, nutrition, and fitness training have made it possible for over forty, over fifty, and even over sixty-year-old athletes to shine, and even out-perform their younger competitors. Once again, I looked to the accomplishments of others to use for my own inspiration.

Today there are a number of seasoned athletes who impress the world with their abilities and record-breaking performances. Audiences get a special thrill in witnessing an aged athlete pull off a masterful performance. What gives these athletes resilience and enables them to persevere when the odds are against their longevity in sport? Wisdom? Strength? Experience? Confidence? The will to win?

I get such a kick out of seeing the old guys beat the young ones. Forty-nine year old major league pitcher, Jamie Moyer, got his first start during President Reagan's second term. He has played for the Texas Rangers, the Baltimore Orioles, and the Boston Red Sox. For years, people complained that Moyer was too old and lacking in speed and strength. Instead, relying on his guile and the precision of his pitches, Moyer's winning percentage has improved with age. After missing the entire 2011 season due to an elbow injury and reconstructive surgery, he has reemerged to prove that he can still pitch.

In spring training of 2012, Moyer proved that age does not limit growth and improvement. In five games, four of which he was the starting pitcher, Moyer allowed just five earned runs over eighteen innings, and struck out sixteen batters. His hard work paid off when he was chosen over two twenty-something pitchers for a spot in the starting rotation of the Colorado Rockies.

Moyer, in his twenty-fifth season, was grateful for the opportunity to succeed and was willing to put in the time and effort to continue his baseball fairy tale. He confided that if he had not tried this, he would have always wondered if he could have done it. Even at age forty-nine, with his gray-streaked hair, Moyer claimed to feel like an excited kid waiting to find out what he was capable of accomplishing. On April 17, 2012, the aged Moyer became the oldest pitcher to ever win a major league baseball game. His sharpness and experience helped to bring the Colorado Rockies to victory over the San Diego Padres. This was Moyer's 268th win during his nearly quarter of a century career of 689 games. One can only imagine the joy and satisfaction that Moyer must have felt as he defeated the young team of Padres. Six of the Padre team players had not even been born when Moyer made his major league debut in 1986. Jamie Moyer's longevity is truly an inspiration.

Major league baseball had a number of players in the over-forty age bracket that excelled at the sport. At forty-one, New York Yankee relief pitcher, Mariano Rivera, was a member of twelve All Star teams, as well as five victorious World Series teams. Rivera's dependable, steady, pitching in the later innings has sealed his reputation as the greatest closer in Major League Baseball history. His teammate, Alex Rodriguez, has described Rivera as "the greatest weapon in baseball."

At the time of his retirement in 2012, forty-five year old Toronto Blue Jay, Omar Vizquel was the only signed player from the 1980s era, and the oldest short stop in major league history. Vizquel won eleven Golden Glove awards, and in 2006, he was the oldest player to win one at age thirty-nine. In 2009, Vizquel became the all-time leader in base hits by a Venezuelan player. He said that he did not want to be sitting at home watching television while he was still able to play at the highest level in the game.

At the Beijing Olympic Games in 2008, forty-one year old Dara Torres became the oldest female swimmer to ever compete in the Olympics. Perhaps the fastest female swimmer in America, Torres was a blink away from a gold medal when she lost the fifty-meter freestyle race by one one-hundredth of a second. A heart-breaking loss, but an astonishing achievement, as it had been eight years since her last Olympics, and retirement from competitive swimming. Launching this comeback, as a new mother, amazed and captured the hearts of all, as Torres was awarded three silver medals.

In 2009, *Sports Illustrated* named Torres as one of the top female athletes of the decade, and at the seventeenth annual ESPY Awards, she won the Best Comeback award. Torres has had surgeries on both shoulders, along with reconstructive knee surgery in 2009, which led to speculation that her swim career was over. In spite of the wear and tear on her body, Torres began training for the 2012 Olympic Games. She hoped to become the oldest Olympic swimmer of all time. In order to clench the individual gold medal that slipped through her fingers in 2008, Torres knew that she would have to surpass athletes who are half her age.

Since 1984, Dara Torres has competed in all but the 1996 and 2004 summer Olympic Games, and she was hoping to end her career with a sixth trip to the Olympics. Torres has said that her drive to compete comes from perseverance and her love of the sport, rather than a need to add to her twelve Olympic medals. Unfortunately, Torres failed to make the 2012 Olympic team, finishing fourth in the qualifying fifty-meter freestyle final. Giving an incredible performance, Torres was outpaced over the final meters. She narrowly missed fulfilling her dream by only nine-hundredths of a second. Although disappointed, Torres knew that she had given it her all. She was happy that at age forty-five she was able to hang in there, placing fourth against girls who were half her age.

Fifty-three year old French racing cyclist, Jeannie Longo did compete in the 2012 London Olympics. Like other vintage athletes, Longo was already competing in the 1984 Olympics before most of her current competitors were born. Considered one of the greatest female cyclists of all time, Longo is a thirteen-time world champion. She has excelled in seven Olympic Games, competing in both road and track, and bicycle racing events. Longo's long career has garnered her four Olympic medals and fifty-eight national championship titles. Unable to commit herself to retirement, Longo has continued to make her way back to the competitive arena. She won the Elite Women time trial in the French Road Championships on June 23, 2011. Like other seemingly ageless wonders, Longo believes that there is always something to work on that will improve her performance. She has chosen to focus on leg speed to prepare for her future victories.

Kathy Martin's special talent lay hidden and undiscovered for over forty years. The sixty-year-old distance runner came to show the world what possibilities and capabilities can be expected from an older athlete. Thirty years ago, Kathy was so out of shape that she could not get through a casual, mile-long jog with her husband. Determined to get fit, she started daily runs and gradually increased her distance. Martin rewarded herself with brownies and hot fudge sundaes, which also served as an incentive to continue on with her workouts. Martin's husband encouraged her to enter in some local road races, which she found to be exciting and addictive. After a few wins, Martin sensed that she had an untapped talent, and believed that she could run even faster.

During her thirties, Martin was consumed with duties as a mother and a real estate agent, however, during her pregnancy, she continued to walk five miles daily. Six weeks after childbirth, Martin resumed her training and conditioning schedule. In her late forties, someone encouraged Martin to enter a track meet. After competing in the mile, and 3,000-meter races, Martin was shocked to learn that her times were just a few seconds from the world records. Martin was on her way to becoming one of the most remarkable distance runners in the world. In her late fifties, she broke records in excess of a dozen events. Since her sixtieth birthday, Martin set nine American records and two world records. Martin set a world record for her age group in the 3,000-meter race with a time of eleven minutes, sixteen-and-a-half seconds. In addition, in her sixty to sixty-four age group, she set the world record for 1,500 meters, with a time of five minutes, twelve point two seconds. Kathy Martin continued to set American and world records in the women's over sixty-five age group. One would never have imagined that an attempt at a casual jog thirty-five years ago could lead to the discovery of one of the fastest senior runners in the world.

During the seventies, Diana Nyad was the greatest long distance swimmer in the world. In 1975, the twenty-six year old made national headlines by swimming twenty-eight miles around New York City's island of Manhattan in just under eight hours. In 1978, at age twenty-eight, Nyad made her first attempt to swim one hundred miles from Havana, Cuba to Key West, Florida. She swam inside a steel shark cage, for nearly forty-two hours, but failed short of her goal. Due to strong currents and bad weather, Nyad was able to complete seventy-six miles before doctors advised her to stop.

In 1979, Nyad set a world record for the longest swim in history as she stroked a 102 miles in open water without a shark cage or a wetsuit. This twenty-seven and one-half hour record, on her thirtieth birthday, was to be Nyad's last competitive swim. Nyad was inducted into the United States' National Women's Sports Hall of Fame in 1986, as well as the International Swimming Hall of Fame in 2003.

Nyad did not swim a single stroke for thirty-one years, although she continued to test her physical endurance with things like hundred mile bike rides and long periods of resisting thirst. As Nyad approached sixty, she felt full of regret. Nyad started swimming again and once again found a desire to train and chase the dream that had eluded her in her prime. Nyad felt that her endurance could be even better at sixty, than at thirty, because her body was almost as strong and she had a better mind.

In August of 2011, Nyad once again attempted the swim from Cuba to Florida. She had to abort her swim after fifty-one miles and twenty-eight hours due to a twelve-hour long asthma attack. A month later, Nyad made a second attempt that came with worse consequences. She incurred multiple Portuguese man-of-war and jellyfish stings. Their toxic venom temporarily left Nyad partially paralyzed, which made breathing stressful. Another attempt in 2012 also ended is disappointment. Nyad refused to give up her dream, and at age sixty-four, she successfully made the Cuba to Florida swim in fifty-three hours in early September of 2013.

Nyad is four decades older than Australian swimmer Susie Maroney, who completed the swim in 1997 at age twenty-two. Nyad aspired to be the first swimmer to complete the feat without a protective shark cage. Nyad admitted to being a bit afraid, but she was determined to overcome the pressure and make it. She was determined to show the world that all dreams are attainable. And that she did. Her mantra during that epic swim was "Find a Way," and with perseverance and persistence, she did just that.

Seventy-one year old, Japanese equestrian, Hiroshi Hoketsu was the oldest Olympian in the 2012 Olympic Games (and the oldest Olympian in the last ninety-two years). That Olympic performance was forty-eight years after his Olympic debut in Tokyo as a twenty-three-year-old show jumper who placed fortieth. At age thirty-five, Hoketsu switched to Dressage because it became too difficult for his eyes to precisely judge the distances to jumps at the high speed required in show jumping.

In 2008, Hoketsu competed at the Beijing Olympics; he placed ninth in team Dressage and thirty-fifth in individual Dressage. His qualification for the 2012 Olympics, with his fifteen-year-old mare, Whisper, was sealed after an unexpected victory at a competition in France early in 2012. Hoketsu had nearly given up on this Olympic dream, as Whisper had been sidelined with tendonitis during most of the previous year. Feeling lucky, Hoketsu credits Whisper's miraculous recovery to a great veterinarian.

Dressage, sometimes referred to as equestrian ballet, is a discipline that requires brains as well as brawn. A rider must possess perfectionist skills, along with rigorous physical discipline, core strength, and balance. Hoketsu's work ethic included a rigorous exercise routine with two daily, hour-long stretching sessions, along with fitness training, and muscle toning exercises. Having ridden horses for nearly sixty years,

Hoketsu considered being in the saddle as natural as walking. Although competitive, Hoketsu's biggest motivation was not competition. A lifetime love of horses and the pursuit of perfection was the driving force behind his dream as he stated:

"As long as I feel as if I'm getting better, that I'm riding better than yesterday, that's the secret. And I do. I honestly believe I'm better today at seventy, than when I was forty."

Hoketsu claimed that age does not matter. He never thought about how old he felt. He found it funny that in 1964, as a twenty-three-year-old show jumper in his home Tokyo Olympics, nobody even noticed him. Surprisingly, forty-eight years later, a circus of camera crews from all over the world showed up at his home calling him a miracle.

Feeling perplexed, Hoketsu claimed: "People say I'm a miracle, but I'm just an ordinary man."

Hoketsu's 2012 Olympic Grand Prix Dressage score of 68.72 was quite respectable, however, it was not up to the level of the top contenders. Unfortunately, in 2016, Hoketsu missed out on qualifying for the Olympics when his horse was taken ill.

If you had a hard time believing there could be an Olympic equestrian who is a septuagenarian, then you would likely not be able to fathom an international gymnastics star that is nonagenarian. Ninety-one year old Johanna Quaas was a former gym teacher and handball champion when she began her gymnastics training at age thirty. More than fifty years later, in 2012, according to Guinness World Records, Quaas was declared the oldest gymnast in the world at eighty-six years old. Quaas has proven that gymnastics is not a sport for only the very young. Not many thirty-year-olds possess the physique, balance, arm strength, and flexibility of Johanna Quaas. She claims to stay young by taking naps and eating a mostly plant-based diet.

Johanna Quaas has said, "My face is old but my heart is young. Maybe the day I stop doing gymnastics is the day I die."

In 2017, the ninety-one year old showed off her incredible moves on the parallel bars on Steve Harvey's television show *Little Big Shots: Forever Young*.

Eighty-one year old Ernestine Shepherd became the world's oldest competitive female body-builder. Riding her bicycle at age eleven, Ernestine was hit by a car, which resulted in a broken ankle. From then on, Ernestine had no interest in exercise and admittedly became a couch potato. Her only goal was to look nice and be noticed, so she just sat pretty and remained inactive for the next forty-five years.

At age fifty-six, Ernestine and her older sister, Mildred, went to the mall to buy swimsuits. After seeing their reflections in the dressing room mirror, the sisters found themselves unhappy with how their bodies had changed over the years. They started taking aerobics classes and later added weight lifting for toning. People started to notice the stunning, muscular sisters, and they were sought out to talk at fitness classes and fashion shows. Sister Mildred dreamed of competing in bodybuilding shows, and one day making history in the Guinness World Records book. Sadly, a brain aneurysm took Mildred's life, which caused Ernestine to sink into a deep depression. She lost her faith, along with her desire to workout.

Five years later Ernestine Shepherd laced up her tennis shoes and made a commitment to fulfill her sister's dream. Ernestine eventually began training with Yohnnie Shambourger, who had won the gold medal in bodybuilding at the Pan American Games, as well as the title of Mr. Universe in 1995. After the age of sixty, Ernestine Shepherd has completed nine marathons and claimed victory in two bodybuilding contests. She fulfilled her sister's dream and was named the Guinness World Records oldest competitive female bodybuilder in 2016 and 2017.

Currently, Shepherd teaches body sculpting at a gym near Baltimore. Known for her signature six-pack abs, Shepherd contends that age is nothing but a number. People in her classes cannot keep up with Ernestine, because they do not have the discipline to reach her fitness level. Shepherd wakes up at three o'clock a.m. for daily runs totaling eighty miles per week. She turns down chocolate cake and settles for bland chicken, along with the bodybuilder's drink of liquid egg whites.

After learning of the accomplishments of these remarkable athletes, I became convinced that age really is just a number. An athlete's body does not give out at a certain age. It is possible for an athlete to become wiser, stronger, and more skilled with age. Age does not restrict an athlete from dreaming new dreams and reaching new goals. Exceptional athletes have a will deep inside them, along with a strong desire to create a vision and follow their dream.

## Exceptional Athletes Have Special Qualities

1. Dedication toward a quest for personal best
2. Motivation to test themselves and develop their best skills
3. Discipline to train hard and maintain strength
4. Persistence to keep trying in spite of injuries and setbacks
5. Commitment to living the dream

## Chapter 15

# What Is the One Thing You Should Never Say to a Dancer?

*There was a man who complained because he had no shoes until he met a man who had no feet*

**—Anonymous**

One thing you should never say to a dancer is: "You will never dance again." Why not? Because it is likely that the spirit within that dancer will defy the odds, prove you wrong, and make you a fool.

All of us can learn about the strength of the human spirit by studying the heart and drive of fallen dancers. If you are faced with a challenging situation, and find yourself wallowing in self-pity, look at those who have been dealt a far worse hand than you. When faced with physical challenge, or tragedy, dancers seem to have a supernatural drive to fight back, to be the dancer they were always meant to be. A dancer's heart will never die; the dancer will always find a way to get back to the dance floor. It might be a different presentation, but the desire to survive, conquer the challenge, and express the dance again will triumph. There is an Indian proverb that sums it all up: "To watch us dance is to hear our hearts speak."

Having witnessed what other dancers have endured, conquered, and achieved, made me laugh at the smallness of my own challenge. If Dr. Wise knew of the spirit of dancers and what they have achieved after tragedy, he would have been embarrassed to tell me that I would never dance again, after a simple hip replacement surgery. There are people who are out there dancing with bodies that have gone through severe trauma. They are once again performing mind-blowing feats in spite of extreme physical limitations. I think Dr. Wise needs to get out more, take his nose out of the textbooks and research, and have a look at the human spirit. Did he really think that replacing my deteriorated hip joint with a nice, new titanium part would keep me from dancing again? I feel as though my new titanium hip joint is actually an enhancement, and an added strength to my dancing.

As I look at the achievements of other dancers who have fought their way back to the dance floor after devastating physical trauma or illness, I feel humbled, mesmerized, and in awe of these miraculous individuals. I have watched their performances with a dropped jaw and tears in my eyes. High-level dancing requires such a high degree of mental concentration and physical control. Mastering the technical and performance skills of high-level dancing is extremely difficult, complicated, and challenging enough for those of us who are healthy, and have two arms and two legs. Instead of pitying ourselves and making excuses for our limitations, we can gain confidence and strength from those who are more challenged than ourselves.

George Velazquez had a life full of dancing and performing. He also found joy and pride as a dance teacher. In 1994, a tragic auto accident changed this dancer's life forever. Doctors had to amputate his left leg, leaving Velazquez full of despair. At age forty-two, his spirit was crushed, and Velazquez lost his identity as a dancer. Depression led to weight gain, and he became bloated and out of shape. Velazquez's dance students missed him and needed him. They scolded their teacher for wasting time with self-pity, while wasting away in the bed, and in the wheelchair. The students encouraged their fallen mentor to get off of his butt and take action. When Velazquez once again tried on one of his expensive dance costumes, and was unable to button it, he made a commitment to educate himself about life and options for amputees. He discovered a desire to give reassurance, understanding, and motivation to other amputees. Years of dance training enabled Velazquez to accelerate his recovery. His dancer's awareness of using the core of his body, and center of balance, helped him to walk on his new prosthesis. Velazquez triumphed over tragedy as he went on to compete against able-bodied professional dancers. I watched a video of George Velazquez dancing with no prosthesis, but a crutch instead. While dancing, he tossed the crutch aside, and danced on one leg! Wow! This was a mind-blowing thing to witness, as most dancers encounter balance issues with two legs. For excellence in teaching, Velazquez won three prestigious Golden Apple awards. This dancer kicked despair in the gut, and went on to dance again, and make a difference in people's lives.

A police motorcycle hit Heather Mills as she walked across a street in 1993. With an injured pelvis, punctured lung, and leg amputated below the knee, Heather's main goal was merely to walk again. She wanted to serve as an example for other amputees by showing them that they could go on to enjoy life again. After the loss of her leg, Heather went back to modeling, and also became a human activist. While delivering one of her speeches, Heather captured the heart of Beetle Paul McCartney. Their five-year marriage ended with a painful split and divorce in 2007.

Heather had become universally disliked over the years, and was aching to change her negative reputation in the eyes of the public. If not a joke, signing up for the television show *Dancing with the Stars* seemed like it would be a huge mistake, for this one-legged dancer. Audiences had witnessed seasons of stars struggling with the stamina, timing, and technique of the show's many difficult dance routines. Ballroom dancing produces impact, weight, and stress on a dancer's legs. Dancing even requires strong feet in order to move one's body away from the standing leg, to produce movement and weight transfer to the other leg. How could a dancer cope with all of that on a prosthetic leg and foot?

I really did not believe it was possible for Heather Mills to cope with this challenge when I heard her name announced as one of the contestants for *Dancing with the Stars*. Like many, I expected that Mills would be the first celebrity to get voted off of the show. I was completely shocked as Mills went on to amaze the audience and stun the judges with good, solid, athletic dancing. She did a mambo routine during week two that was absolutely spellbinding. Mills showed energetic, Cuban hip action, which is not easily produced by novice dancers, and she nailed a tricky back walkover in the middle of the routine. If I had not witnessed it with my own eyes, I would not have believed it was possible.

Judge Carrie Ann Inaba was really shocked as she remarked, "What in the world? I'm just blown away by you. The level of difficulty in that routine was far higher than anyone else's routine tonight. You nailed it!"

Judge Bruno Tonioli was mystified by Mills' dancing performance as he exclaimed, "You nailed it! Beyond any expectation! Red Hot, Heather. I can't believe it!"

I witnessed another show-stealing performance from a one-legged dancer in the Cirque du Soleil show, *Michael Jackson, The Immortal World Tour*. Break-dancer, Jean Sok amazed the audience with his astonishing athletic ability on crutches. It was hard for me to take my eyes off of him as he danced, spun around, and even did the moon walk on crutches. Certainly when Jean Sok lost his leg, he could not have imagined that he would eventually be inspiring audiences worldwide with his heart-stealing performances.

One of the most emotional dancing comebacks ever has to be that of Richard "Steelo" Vazquez. This top professional street dancer, choreographer, actor, and performance artist suffered a brain aneurysm in 2011. Close to dying, Vasquez spent nine weeks in intensive care during his six months of recovery in the hospital. Vazquez had to learn to walk and speak again as the dancer within yearned to get back to his place as a member of the dance group, The Groovaloos. Challenging himself, Vasquez fought through physical rehabilitation, five days a week, seven hours a day. On May 1, 2012, "Steelo" performed with The Groovaloos on *Dancing with the Stars*, on live television, in front of millions of viewers. I watched this performance with tears running down my cheeks.

I remembered my college friend who had a brain aneurysm one day, and fell dead right on the spot. Another friend of mine suffered a brain aneurysm, never recovered, and lived in a nursing home for several years until he died. I was absolutely dumbfounded by Steelo's performance. The bravery, the passion, and the fight back against overwhelming odds, was incredible. Of course, Steelo's standard of performance was not back to the high level it had once been, but I have no doubt that it will get there, in the not too distant future. Richard "Steelo" Vazquez is truly a dancing miracle.

Do you think that being confined to a wheelchair could stop a dancer from dancing? Hardly. Wheelchair ballroom dancing began in 1972, and has become a very popular sport throughout the world. There are wheelchair couple dances, where each of the two partners is in a wheelchair. Another classification consists of a couple, with one partner in a wheelchair, while the other able-bodied partner is standing. Having seen a few of these routines performed was a heart-warming experience. You just cannot imagine what a beautiful thing it is until you see it.

There is also a group wheelchair division, where four, six, or eight couples, dance in formation. Any dance can be danced with a partner in a wheelchair—the Waltz, the Foxtrot, the Cha Cha, and even the Hustle. In addition to being enjoyed as a social and recreational activity, in over forty countries, wheelchair ballroom dancing is growing as a competitive sport. There are over five thousand registered dancers in Europe, and eight thousand in Asia. Often there are as many as three hundred wheelchair dance competitors at overseas ballroom dancing competitions. Wheelchair ballroom dancing is popular and may very well be a Paralympic sport at sometime in the future.

## What Makes Amazing Dancers

1. The ability to rebound from setbacks. These individuals accept injury or tragedy, deal with it, and move forward.
2. The ability to be realistic in setting a goal.
3. The ability to take action in their own healing.
4. The ability to keep a positive attitude.
5. The ability to take control and commit to workouts and training.

## Chapter 16

# Dance Training Offers Life Lessons

Imitation is not just the sincerest form of flattery—
it's the sincerest form of learning.

**—George Bernard Shaw**

Hotel personnel can easily spot the ballroom dancers amongst crowds of customers meandering through a hotel lobby. The dancers present an attractive picture, composed of good posture and a neat, tidy appearance. You will likely never see a male dancer schlepping around in public wearing a baggy T-shirt, cargo shorts, flip flops, and a backpack. Sadly, the latter seems to be an accepted uniform for the general American population. Just have a look around the next time you walk through an airport or a shopping mall.

Anyone can pick up some helpful hints by observing a dancer's overall appearance and behavior. A few minor changes and additions to an average person's basic presentation can be life enhancing, as well as improve the way one is perceived and received by others. Think of the more favorable impression those cargo-geared, backpack toting individuals would present if they merely lost the back weight, and went to a nice roller-bag. How much better would they look if they stood up tall, threw their shoulders back, and put on a nice fitting shirt and pair of pants or jeans? A nice belt and pair of shoes would add some polish and upgrade a guy's overall look. With a few inexpensive upgrades, those guys might even draw in some interested looks from the opposite sex. Generally, women are not attracted to slovenly men who wear flip-flops, or those silly, plastic shoes called "Crocs." Beach shoes belong at the beach.

With their fit, trim figures, lady dancers can certainly pull off wearing some hot, trendy outfits; they always seem appropriately dressed for the occasion. It is doubtful that you will see a ballroom lady dressed in an inappropriate or slutty outfit out in public. Sexy costumes are reserved for the competition dance floor. Showtime is Showtime; practice time is taken seriously for learning and training by most ballroom dancers. Serious dancers do not show up for practice sessions wearing tight, short dresses, bustiers, or tube tops. A serious dancer wears comfortable clothing that stays in place and enables her to move around and use her body to produce the athletic movement required for dancing.

A dancer's hair is every bit as important as clothing, in both formal and informal situations. An unraveling hairdo or a hairpiece that falls off is certain to be a turn off to competition judges. Even during a dance lesson, long, stringy, unsecured hair is not only a distraction to the student, but an annoyance to the teacher as well. A neat, tied back hairdo would be advice well heeded by a serious student of any sporting endeavor.

I once had a riding instructor who refused to teach a student who showed up with her hair blowing around in her eyes, as she rode her horse. He insisted that hair always be tied back or tucked up under the riding helmet. How could one possibly be able to concentrate on a game of golf, tennis, hockey, lacrosse, soccer, or volleyball with hair blowing across one's face, blocking the view?

Years ago, young tennis phenom sisters, Venus and Serena Williams, were proud to display their beaded hairdos. After being fined for beads that came loose, and spilled onto the competition court, the sisters came to realize that their trendy look brought about negative consequences. Wild, unruly hair can be an unwelcome distraction to officials, competitors, and audiences as well. It is a sign of disrespect to coaches, and shows a lack of serious commitment on the part of the athlete.

In life, as in dancing, you only have a moment to make a first impression. All of us would like to be judged by what is on the inside, but unfortunately, we live in a visually influenced society. In a job interview or sales presentation, your efforts toward a neat appearance will likely be appreciated and rewarded. In addition, by taking a few extra minutes to make yourself look good, you will also feel good about yourself. If you look good, you feel good.

Being healthy, fit, and trim is a way of life for most ballroom dancers. It takes energy and strength to produce movement for good dancing. Stamina is essential for many rounds of dancing that are required at a competition. Obviously, there is no place for recreational drugs or cigarettes in the life of a serious competitive dancer. In addition, a healthy diet and body maintenance are essential elements to the life of a high-level dancer. I believe Jack Lalanne got it right when he said, "Exercise is King, nutrition is Queen, put them together, and you've got a kingdom."

Women dancers know that they will be wearing form-fitting ball gowns, and skimpy Latin costumes, thus they live in fear of showing unwanted jiggles or rolls of fat. Men dancers as well, do not want to show bellies or love handles under their skintight Lycra slacks and shirts. Nobody wants to see flesh spilling over the top of a dancer's waistband. The "muffin top" look is not flattering.

In addition to giving people the incentive to dress attractively, and maintain a fit, healthy body, ballroom dancing teaches one manners, memorization skills, and performance skills. Social dancing teaches etiquette that would be a benefit to all. Men learn how to treat a lady by offering an extended hand to ask for a dance, pulling out her chair, and opening doors. A lady learns to respond graciously to invitations. People learn to become socially engaging, which builds communication skills and confidence.

Hey guys, women are attracted to men who can dance. You do not have to be the best looking, or even the best dancer. If a guy can dance reasonably well, he will get dates.

> A man who knows how to dance
> can make any woman feel good.
> **—Barbara Haller**

Memorization skills come into play as dancers learn sequences of dance steps. Such groupings are applied to the skill level of the partner with whom one happens to be dancing. Obviously, advanced students are capable of more complex material than a beginner who has just learned the basics. In a social setting, the more experienced dancer learns to dance down to the level of a less experienced partner. Ballroom dancing enables people with different backgrounds and skill levels to interact with each other. Similarly, in business, employees from different departments with varying skill levels must learn to interact in a cohesive manner.

Competition dancers learn performance skills and the pursuit of excellence. They walk out onto the dancer floor with posture and confidence. They learn how to perform, show their skills, and entertain an audience, as they show the character of each particular dance, whether it be a Tango with fire and attitude, or a flirty Rumba.

Dancers learn to share and be respectful of others. Social dancers are expected to change partners often at dances. Some dancers are more experienced, skilled, personable, and fun to dance with, thus are more in demand as a partner by other dance attendees. No one's time should be monopolized, and each dancer learns to try to share time with several partners throughout the evening.

In Pro Am competition dancing, a professional teacher might be competing with quite a few amateur students (sometimes more than ten) at one, four-to-five day competition. With all of the different divisions and age categories, that teacher could be dancing in a few hundred, one-minute-fifteen-second heats over a few days. Some of those heats have a semi-final, and then a final round. Big multi-dance scholarship events might have four rounds of dancing. Often, such a teacher could be dancing with his many students from early morning, until after midnight with very few rest periods or breaks throughout the day. The students must be respectful of their teacher's physical exertion, and also learn to be sharing, and self-sufficient regarding warm up, and practice time.

Whether a ballroom dancer is sharing social dance partners or a professional competition teacher, he or she must learn to share the partner's time with others. The teacher is not a mechanical practice machine there to serve the needs of only one student. Ballroom dancers learn that the whole world does not revolve around them as an individual. One must take some personal responsibility in his or her own advancement. A good dance student cannot simply rely on the dance teacher to make him or her a better dancer. Similarly, an employee of a company cannot expect the boss to do all the work in order to make that employee become more skilled or accomplished. Whether you are an employee, a musician, a writer, an athlete, or a dancer, you must make the effort, do the work, and put in the hours to reap the benefits and the rewards.

A true champion shows the drive to excel and takes responsibility for his or her own advancement. Some dance students go so far as to learn every count of every step for all of their competition dance routines (which could be as many as 19). Those of us who practice on our own are able to dance all of our routines, on time, to music, and by ourselves. It must surely look odd to onlookers, who see me at the gym, dancing around the aerobics room without a partner, but a dancer has to do what it takes to get to the top.

One thing that dancers learn to develop is a keen sense of spatial awareness. Social dancers and competitors alike must learn to have "floor craft" as they maneuver around a dance floor. When many couples are on a crowded dance floor, dancers learn to follow the "line of dance," which is a conceptual path that is parallel to the edge of the dance floor. Dance couples agree to travel along this line of dance, in a counterclockwise direction, in order to avoid collisions. This concept would be useful at country club dances where I have seen dancing couples actually get into fights after repetitively bumping into each other.

Apparently, most pedestrians have no clue about spatial awareness. The general population would certainly benefit from studying a bit of "floor craft" and using some "line of dance" as they attempt to navigate through pedestrian traffic. Since dancers are trained to be aware of their movement in relation to the presence of others, they always look around before they move or take a step. In addition, dancers tend to follow the natural flow of traffic in an airport, or a shopping mall, which is like following the line of dance. Dancers do not stop in the middle of flowing pedestrian traffic to look in a bag, greet friends, or look up at an airport monitor, thus bringing a halt to traffic flow behind them and causing a pedestrian pile-up.

When exiting a narrow hallway, dancers stay respectfully on the right, so as not to run smack into another person entering the same hallway from the opposite direction. A dancer is not likely to come barging out of a mall store, pushing a stroller, and plow into ongoing walking traffic. A dancer would first look both ways, and then choose a path, and move forward in a straight line. Have you seen people walking in an airport who are oblivious to anyone else's presence? They rudely cut into the paths of others as they walk with their eyes downward while texting on their phones.

Have you ever seen the way many people handle double doors at the entrance to a store or restaurant? Obviously, the intention is for patrons to enter using the door on the right, as those leaving are intended to use the door on the left. It is shocking to see how many people choose to go out the same door on the right, which others are using to try to enter the store. Not only is that against the "line of dance," but also it is against common sense and respect for others.

Ballroom dancing offers a new sense of purpose in the lives of many. Initially, many people who stumble into a ballroom dance studio are feeling insignificant, bored with their lives, or lonely. Often, a wife brings her husband in kicking and screaming. Time and time again, I have witnessed the husbands get hooked on the dance lessons. Surprisingly, it is often the men who want to keep coming back for more learning.

I have noticed that ballroom dancing becomes a big thing for many women who are empty nesters, do not play sports, or do not have a major hobby taking up their free time. Many women want to take private lessons nearly every day. Some become obsessed turn into "dance monsters." They want to take more lessons than the teacher is able to accommodate. These women become demanding and competitive with other students for the teacher's attention. A dance monster student will eventually learn that she is not the center of the Universe, and she will learn one of life's basic lessons—sharing.

Even if you have no interest in ballroom dancing, simply emulating the ways of a dancer can be a positive influence on your life. You will end up thinking more about your appearance: your clothing, your posture, and your hair. You will be able to walk into a party, a job interview, or a blind date with poise and confidence. Giving up smoking and adopting a healthy diet will make you feel great.

If you decide to actually become a ballroom dancer, you will learn skills that will help you navigate a social dance venue. You will improve your skills in social interaction, memorization, and performance. You will learn to be conscious of your own spatial awareness, to be respectful of others, and to negotiate pedestrian traffic, whether you are dancing or just walking in public. Ballroom dancing might enhance your life in ways that you have never imagined. You just might find a new spark in your marriage or a new zest for life!

## Darla's Favorite Health Drink

Walking into an airport one day, I spotted one of my all-time idols, Jack Lalanne, sitting right there in front of me on a bench all by himself. He was about ninety-two years old at the time, and this was about four years before his death. I ran over and introduced myself to Jack and told him how I remembered watching his television show, and that my mother and I would do exercises in front of our black and white television when I was about five-years old. I fondly recalled the jumpsuit that Jack wore, which emphasized his wide shoulders and narrow hips. As a dog-crazy kid at the time, I always looked forward to seeing Jack's beautiful white German shepherds come running onto the set at the end of the show.

I told Jack that forty-five years ago, my mom had purchased one of his rubber exercise bands, and I had just recently purchased The Jack Lalanne Power Juicer. I explained that as a ballroom dancer, I was on a quest to achieve maximum health and strength. Jack's face lit up as he told me that his mission was to turn America onto juicing. He cautioned me to never eat anything that comes out of a box because processed foods are the cause of many health problems. Jack wished me luck and told me to keep juicing, because it is the key to a long, healthy life.

For the past few years, my favorite juice drink has been carrot, apple, and ginger. I usually just throw in five or six carrots, a couple of apples, and about an inch of ginger root. Of course, it can be adjusted to add more carrots and fewer apples, or vice versa. I never thought I would like vegetable juice, but the sweetness of the apple, and the bite of the ginger, makes the overall taste of this combination absolutely delicious.

Recently, I made another version of this drink, substituting kale for the carrots. I shoved about six or seven giant kale leaves into the juicer, along with the apples, and ginger. The rich, green drink comes out looking like pond scum, more suited for tadpoles and turtles than for drinking. Looks are deceiving. I kid you not—the taste is fabulous! I am convinced that apples and ginger can make anything taste great.

# Chapter 17

# What Makes or Breaks a Winning Performance?

*Adversity causes some men to break; others to break records.*
**—William Arthur Ward**

How does an athlete or a dancer develop the mental toughness and emotional control to lay down a winning performance? Despite having the most talent, the best training, and the most experience, even the most favored athletes have failed under pressure. The pressure to perform causes performance anxiety, which is often referred to as choking.

Similar to stage fright in a musician or actor, athletes who choke are unable to perform routine tasks as their bodies become tense, and they lose their touch, fluidity of movement, and concentration. We have all watched the world's best miss a free throw, a short putt, or an easy drop shot over the net. Some athletes go into panic mode, which causes them to stop thinking or lose their memory.

Why do the best athletes often choke? During the mid-1990s, Greg Norman, the "Great White Shark," was considered by many to be the greatest golfer in the world. In spite of his talent, Norman constantly buckled under pressure during major tournaments. Known as one of the worst choke artists of all-time, Norman's 1996 Masters loss has been considered the worst moment in golf history. Entering the final day of the tournament, with a six-stroke lead over Nick Faldo, Norman fell apart and shot a seventy-eight, while Faldo shot a sixty-seven. Faldo won by five strokes to claim the coveted green jacket. It was probably one of the saddest sports losses of all time as everyone from the spectators, to the officials, and even his opponent, felt Norman's pain. What caused Greg Norman to choke at crucial moments of tournaments? Was he thinking that it was such a slam-dunk that he got too relaxed? Did he lose his focus?

In the world of figure skating, Michelle Kwan has been considered one of the world's most talented. With five world championships and nine U.S. titles, Kwan still failed to win Olympic gold. Kwan let her nerves get the best of her and choked at two consecutive Olympics, each time giving up the gold to a newer, less talented competitor. Her first disappointment was at Nagano Olympics in 1998. After winning the world and U.S. championships, Kwan was the reigning queen of her sport. Unfortunately, she failed to show her usual brilliance as she skated safely and conservatively. Kwan's performance lacked risk and energy. She was unable to open up and let herself skate freely, without fear and tension. On the other hand, Kwan's teenage challenger, Tara Lipinski, dazzled the judges and spectators with her sheer joy of skating. Lipinski nailed her performance, winning gold, displaying all of the qualities that were missing in Kwan's silver medal performance.

Four years later in Salt Lake City, Kwan once again came to the Games favored to win. As the four-time world champion, it seemed as though the judges were dying to give Kwan the gold. For the second time this most talented skater self-destructed. Kwan's performance was cautious and tight, resulting in a fall in her long program. A déjà vu moment ensued as another presumably less talented American teenager blissfully skated her way to the gold, leaving a disappointed Kwan holding the bronze medal. Who can explain the self-sabotage of this most talented and revered skater? Was Michelle Kwan overconfident? Was she lacking in aggression and self-control? Did the pressure of performing rob Kwan of her joy for skating?

Ballroom dancing competitions are similar to figure skating in that the joyful, energetic, yet relaxed performer is often victorious over the subdued, yet more talented and technically proficient competitor. A contestant who portrays relaxation and happiness captivates judges and audiences.

There are so many talented ballroom dancers, who like Michelle Kwan, have what it takes to win the big one, but fail to put it all together and thus never reach their potential. Recently, I was watching a retired pro dancer competing with students in the Pro Am division. His dancing was technically stellar, and he had such a charismatic quality about him. Curiously, I inquired why this guy was never a champion, and why he didn't just find a good partner and go back to professional competition? I was told that Mr. Charisma had had several good partners over the years, but he "never got along with them." Afside from that, I was told that Mr. Charisma was just not a good performer. I know that a lot of pro dancing couples fight like cats and dogs, but how could that great dancing guy not be a good performer? I have seen him dancing out on the competition floor with his students looking so happy, energetic, and fabulous. He sure looked like a great performer to me.

That is exactly right, I was told. The pressure is off now, because he is not out there dancing for a big, important, championship. He is just kicking back and having fun with his students. Aha. That is it! No pressure equals a great performance. So often, we hear about a dance student, or athlete, who puts out an awesome performance in practice sessions, and then loses it in competition. Why do many of these athletes and dancers choke and fail, and eventually quit and give up? Which ones gave it all up, when they were just around the corner from breaking through to victory? What would have happened if they had found a way to overcome failure and unleash the winning performance within?

Michael Jordan once said, "I've missed more than nine thousand shots in my career. I've lost almost three hundred games. Twenty-six times, I've been trusted to take the game winning shot and missed. I've failed over, and over, and over again in my life. And that is why I succeed."

Why are many athletes so afraid to fail? If only they could realize that failure is not fatal. It is only temporary. Does anyone remember Michael Jordan for all of those shots that he missed and the games that he lost? No, people remember Michael Jordan for the great athlete that he was and all of the games that he won. Michelle Kwan will not be remembered for her Olympic losses. Fans and experts will remember her as the most talented and most decorated figure skater in U.S. history.

Whatever the causes may be for one's past failures, one must avoid shame and learn to recover and move forward. A true champion will learn to stop, analyze, and then take control of a situation that is spinning out of control. One can develop the tools to help one's self get back on track, after or even during a meltdown.

I remember an event in 2006 when I counseled myself out of a major meltdown. I was able to use my sports psychology training to meet every destructive hurdle with a positive counter action.

After a successful year of competition as an intermediate level dancer, I was selected to perform an exhibition dance with Jim at the prestigious Ohio Star Ball competition. The big evening of professional competitions, along with youth and amateur honor dance presentations, was going to be co-hosted by actress Marilu Henner and be televised.

Jim and I had been practicing my Foxtrot/Cha Cha medley routine for a few months. The thought of dancing in front of many thousands of people, on national television, was both exciting and frightening. Striving to make our dance routine worthy of the upcoming honor led to some tense practice sessions. There was a point after the Foxtrot portion of our routine where I was to rip off my long skirt to reveal a shorter skirt underneath while we changed pace and launched into a lively Cha Cha. We had not realized that the material of the skirt was too stretchy to make the Velcro attachment come undone every time I yanked on it. We tried it so many different ways, but I could not consistently get the job done smoothly. It was causing me great stress and panic, so two days before the event, we decided that Jim would reach around my waist and undo the skirt, during those three seconds when the music changed from one song to another. The burden of that task was off of me, but the stress was still there.

My father had died two weeks before we arrived at the Ohio Star Ball competition. I had to transition from stress and depression, to happiness and relaxation in my performances at the dance competition. I danced pretty well during our first two days of competition. I had a chance to perform the TV routine in the competition the night before the big televised performance. After competing throughout the day, I was feeling tired, and my throat was sore, which reflected in my performance that evening. It went okay until near the end of the routine when I almost tripped myself. I was really bummed because I was favored to win that event and I did not even place in the top three.

The following day was another long day of competition for Jim and all of his students. We were given a scheduled practice time to run through our TV routine in the adjacent arena where the big show would take place later that evening. The producer and the cameramen would be present to plan lighting, camera angles, and such for each performance. When my time slot came up, Jim was still competing with his students and was unable to practice with me. I flipped out. I ran over to the well-known producer, Aida Moreno, and explained that Jim was still competing next door. Remembering my lackluster performance on the previous evening, I was on the verge of tears, as I gave Aida the details.

"I am probably the most inexperienced, lowest level dancer performing here tonight. Nobody needs to practice more than I do!"

Aida tried to calm me down, telling me not to worry, and to just come back with Jim when he was finished competing. My stomach was in knots for another hour. Finally, Jim and I showed up for our practice session. Aida directed us out onto the floor, and we ran through our routine. It went okay, but I would have liked to be able to relax and dance it a few more times.

Aida came over to me and offered some encouraging words. "You don't dance like a beginner. That is a really cute routine."

We had a couple of hours off to relax and regroup before the big event. I could hardly eat any dinner. I was stressed and Jim was exhausted. Soon, we were in our costumes, and back in the arena with the lights, the cameras, and the action. Jim and I were scheduled to do our dance fairly early in the evening, so we went behind the bleachers to practice our routine.

After competing all day with students, and doing probably seven different Cha Cha routines, Jim was blanking out on parts of my routine. I could not blame Jim for being fatigued, but the consequences were causing me some major stress. After making our way over to the on-deck area, we were informed that our performance had to be pushed back because one of the other performing pros was tired and had to be moved to earlier in the schedule so he could get to bed.

*Are you fricken kidding me?*

I was in disbelief and furious. At this point, I was primed for a major meltdown. Jim was already exhausted from doing way more dancing than the prima donna who had to get his beauty sleep. There were ten-year-old kids performing that evening who were more experienced and more accomplished than me. If that were not enough, there was not only a huge audience in front of us, but there were thousands, if not millions of people watching on television, including many of my friends and family. Inside, I was flipping out, as I just sort of stood there and took it all in.

*Calm down. Just calm down,* I told myself. I realized that no one there was going to reach out, hold my hand, and baby me. Yes, I was the baby in this group of performers, but I had to take control of the situation. I had to take the bull by the horns and run this rodeo. I told myself, *I may not be the most experienced, or the best dancer, but we will give a good performance. I am not going to let all of these negative circumstances keep me from showing the best of what I can do, right here, and now.*

Jim and I had lots of extra time so we went behind the bleachers to practice again. I told Jim that if he forgot part of the routine, not to worry, I would lead, and he could follow me. It sounded ridiculous that I was offering to lead one of the world's best, but if he forgot something, I knew I could just keep dancing my part, and he would catch on.

Finally we were back in the on-deck area, and it was about three minutes until we would be walking onto the floor to take our places. I looked over at all of the lights and the cameramen pushing the wheeled cameras up and down the floor. I felt the butterflies in my stomach. I told myself that even if I messed up and tripped myself, and fell down, it would be still be okay because Aida could just edit my routine out of the show. *No pressure, no problem,* I told myself.

At that moment, Mr. Ohio Star Ball himself, the owner and organizer, Sam Sodano, came up behind me and placed his hands on my shoulders. He whispered to me, "You are going to do a great job. Have fun."

That single vote of confidence was all I needed, at that moment, to know that everything was going to be all right.

I had a big smile as we walked out onto the floor and took our starting positions on opposite sides of the floor. The music started, and our Foxtrot was off to Michael Bolton singing, *Fly Me to the Moon.* The dance was going well, and I nailed that pose as Jim came up behind me, tore off my skirt, and threw it across the floor. The audience roared with delight. Into the Cha Cha we sashayed, to Michael Bolton's *Dance with Me*. I was really having fun as we headed down the home stretch. I told myself to stay alert and step deliberately. *I will not allow myself to trip.* Done!

The audience was clapping as we danced off of the floor. *Phew.* What a thrill! That was the best I had ever danced that routine. What a relief that I was able to hold myself together. I immediately ran to find my friend Debbie who had a glass of champagne waiting for me.

 **DARLA'S TIPS FOR**

## Avoiding a Meltdown

1. Prepare yourself well so that you can perform your skills and technique almost automatically and with confidence.
2. Think of your competition as just another practice session.
3. Visualize yourself performing well and being successful.
4. Don't get caught up in thinking about too many little things. Remember the most important things, such as listening to the music, or moving with power.
5. Be positive. Think about winning, not about losing. Don't say, "he's better than me" or "she will win." Say, "I will give a great performance" or "I will win."
6. Calm yourself. Relax, breathe, and think about having fun.
7. Don't dwell on past failures. Nobody wins all of the time. Learn to pump yourself up for the next competition. When I find myself unhappy with my performance, or feeling like I did not receive my just rewards, I like to think of my favorite line from Psalm 30: *Weeping may endure for a night, but joy cometh in the morning.*

# Chapter 18

# Sports Psychology and Dancing

I do not try to dance better than anyone else.
I only try to dance better than myself.

**—Mikhail Baryshnikov**

Sports psychology is one of my favorite topics, but I don't feel that many competitive ballroom dancers have explored it. More than twenty-five years ago, I was fortunate to have studied this topic in a course taught by renowned sports psychologist, Dr. Robert Rotella.

At the time, I was a competitive equestrian. Building confidence and self-esteem can be tough if you always feel that the competition has one up on you, in every aspect of the sport. Competing against the elite, who could afford to buy the finest horses, equipment, clothing, and training, was daunting to say the least.

Imagine the personal head games one encounters, when his or her athletic partner is a twelve-hundred-pound animal. A partner with whom you cannot hold a conversation, nor verbally share thoughts or feelings. A rider's only communication with a horse is through body actions, along with the rider's physical manifestation of his or her state of being, such as calmness, tenseness, passivity, or aggression. Riders experience the same mental issues faced by any athlete: uncertainty, pressure, anxiety, fear, tension, and lack of confidence. There were days when I had great success, and others when I would choke, and mentally self-destruct, which is typical of many athletes.

Sports psychology teaches athletes to overcome the mental hurdles that stand in the way of a great performance. Prior to competition, athletes often experience fear and lack of confidence. During and following a competition, an athlete might feel frustration, self-doubt, jealously, or anger. In sports psychology, we learn techniques that help us to concentrate and gain self-confidence. An athlete can learn how to get over a bad day and achieve consistency in future performances.

One summer course of studying sports psychology with Dr. Rotella transformed and elevated my competitive performances for years to come. The number of my equestrian wins skyrocketed, along with my confidence. Friends started calling me "Starla Darla." I loved it. Some people even made fun of me saying, "Oh, she's got magic sports psychology." I really did not care what anyone said about me. I was winning. They were not. For me, sports psychology was magic; but it was something that any athlete could get, and not at a high price. That one course with one book, and a few private counseling sessions was not high in cost, but certainly high in value.

When I began competing in ballroom dancing competitions, I was able to apply everything that I learned from that sports psychology course to my dancing. Certainly dancers have the advantage of having a language-speaking human being for a partner, rather than a horse that whinnies and snorts.

In the beginning stages of learning any sport, I doubt that any athlete is brimming with confidence and emotional fortitude. I have seen adult dancers behave in ways that are surprisingly immature, ridiculous, and pathetic. Some dancers are so concerned with winning that they lose their focus and become irrational. They have so many head games going on that they are not doing what they are there to do—dance! Jim has often told me about various students, who after a very strong practice session, have gone out to the competition floor and "just lost it." I have witnessed nerve-induced whining and crying, along with negative commentary about the other contestants. Dance students have said things like, "I'm so much better than she is!" and, "How could those judges place that fat lady above me?" In reality, the overweight dancer had fantastic energy, animation, and better technique than the whiny complainer who looked tense and restrained as she danced.

I have often suggested to these ladies that they study a bit of sports psychology. Never once have any of them accepted that my suggestion was worth pursuing. Most of these highly competitive women are of the mindset that more training, plus massive quantities of lessons, equals victory. Some even believe that an alcoholic beverage will calm their nerves and make them dance better. Sadly, it seems as though these women, as athletes, are missing the most important element of competition, which is the development of one's mental attitude.

How often have we heard golfer, Jack Nicklaus, quoted as saying: "The game of golf is 90% mental and 10% physical." Following that thought, as dancers, we wonder why the winner of a particular ballroom dance event is not always the best technical dancer of the group. Often, the winner who lacks in technique exudes confidence, comfort, and sheer joy of being out there on the dance floor. It is possible for all levels of talent to make it to the top. A lesser talented athlete can create motivation and confidence through his or her own thinking. Qualities of patience and persistence can be used as an edge over competitors. Everyone has fears and doubts. Some convince themselves they have no chance of being successful, and concentrate on negative thoughts like who might beat them in the competition. A winner walks out to the competition with the feeling that he or she can beat anybody.

I have known many dancers who have an internal battle. They are not willing to be brave enough to show commitment to being a winner. They make up all kinds of reasons as to why they did not dance well. I have heard quite an array of excuses such as, I did not get enough sleep the night before the competition, or I did not get to eat what I wanted beforehand, or my events were scheduled too late at night, or I am too short, and all of the better dancers are tall. One lady even confided in me that she did not dance well at a competition because she was unable to have a bowel movement in the morning, before she danced. I do sympathize with these excuses, because we all have internal fears and struggles. I am sure that there are hundreds of us dancers who feel like we are going to pee in our pants as we walk out onto a big competition floor. All of us must learn to win the battle within ourselves.

There are many skilled ballroom dancers who are just not good competitors. They either have compatibility issues with their partners, or perhaps are unable to perform under pressure. A little bit of sports psychology training can be so beneficial to competitive dancers. I believe many dancers miss their potential or even moments of greatness, because they just cannot get a grip on the mental side of competing. A true champion develops the maturity and self-control to address negative issues and eliminate the excuses. For example, if a morning bowel movement is necessary for a particular individual to produce a good dancing performance, then that dancer should think about waking up a half-hour earlier in the morning and treating herself to a bowl of raisin bran and a cup of coffee. It is not rocket science.

In ballroom dancing, it can take several years for an individual to develop the maturity and skills it takes to win at the highly competitive, top level of dancing. So many ballroom students quit dancing because they want quick results and instant gratification. They are simply not willing to do the work it takes to develop their minds as well as their physical skills. They cop out, because they are not willing to make a commitment to being a winner. It is too easy to give in, or give up, and make excuses.

Dancers, like other athletes, must learn to develop courage and learn to turn pressure into power. They must learn to concentrate on happiness and motivation. You can learn to think like a winner, or you can think like a loser. Only you can take control of your emotions.

Once you win the battle within yourself, and gain emotional fortitude, you will feel empowered, and that will give you a tremendous edge over your competition. I laugh, as I recall one particular lady who I danced against in my intermediate days. I thought that she was such a graceful, lovely dancer, and in some ways better than myself. My competitor always showed such nervousness in the on-deck area before we went out to dance our events. I observed her, as I was wandering around or warming myself up in the corner. I could sense that the mere sight of me was upsetting to her, as I casually practiced a few steps. This opponent would get herself so worked up that I could see the worried look in her eyes, as she was just standing there next to her teacher.

As the months marched on, I became more confident, and this particular lady became more of a basket case. About a year later, we were at the Emerald Ball, one of the biggest competitions of the year. Once again, I was warming up near the on-deck area, and the same old scenario transpired once again. My competitor looked so stressed as she eyeballed my relaxed, confident air. I saw her teacher put his hands on her shoulders, and force her to turn around and face him, so as not to look at me! I have to admit that I felt a sort of sadistic pleasure watching this silent interaction. Who would have thought that I could be so threatening to someone; especially one who I felt might be a better dancer?

At this competition, we danced in eight single dance events, so we danced the Waltz, Tango, Foxtrot, and Viennese Waltz twice. There were only three judges for these early-in-the day heats, and they awarded first, second, and third placements in each dance. I got nothing! I was clearly one of the best dancers in this group, however, I knew there was some political favoritism going on, and so I was neither surprised nor upset. The situation was predictable. I told Jim that I was happy with my performance, and I looked forward to winning the big scholarship event later in the day. How is that for confidence after getting kicked in the gut? I knew there would be nine or eleven judges on the next judging panel, and the results would be more fair, because the politics would "come out in the wash," as I like to say.

As it turned out, I was the big winner at the end of the day. I really had to credit my success to my study of sports psychology, and the application of its principles and tools. I could have whined and said that the other competitors were better than me, and all of the judges hated me. Or worse, I could have resorted to drinking alcohol, or even scratched my next event. Instead, I maintained my composure, and followed my planned course of action.

The exercises that I learned in the study of sports psychology are beneficial in so many ways. They are confidence building, relaxing, and fun.

I remember one really fun exercise, in particular, that we practiced in Dr. Rotella's Sports Psychology seminar. This exercise will help any athlete to concentrate and control emotions. The exercise begins with the athlete acting out the motion of his or her sport i.e., swinging an imaginary golf club, or a tennis racquet, or dancing around the room. A partner stands beside the athlete and acts out the voice of negative thoughts by shouting out all kinds of annoying and mean phrases at the athlete, such as: "You're such a loser," "Your swing sucks," "You are going to trip and fall down," "Everybody is so much better than you." You can even have your partner throw things at you (like socks), in order to disturb your concentration. This will force the athlete to tune out negative thoughts and other distractions. The athlete learns that the performance is the only thing that matters. Negative and hurtful statements are unwelcome, and have no bearing on the athlete's performance.

Visualization exercises have had such a huge positive impact on my competitive performances, in both the equestrian and dancing arenas. An athlete can use this mental rehearsal to orchestrate and describe the details of an upcoming event. It can be done while you are drinking your coffee, or in a hotel room, or on a plane, while you are taking a walk, while you are at the gym on the elliptical machine, or stationary bike, or sitting in a boring meeting at work (although that would surely not be pleasing to your boss). Years ago, I even used visualization exercises to get through my grandmother's funeral. It was so emotionally painful that I tried to disconnect in order to avoid falling apart. During much of the funeral service, I was jumping my horse around courses of jumps in my head. I had to use this escape to get through the painful event.

There are two ways you can view this mental rehearsal: You can see yourself from the view of a camera (or as another person who is watching your performance), or the other option is to view the performance as you are living it, and feeling what is happening, as it is happening. I like to practice my dance routines using both of these views. I can imagine that I am watching a movie of myself doing every step of every one of my dance routines. I watch myself doing the graceful arm styling, as I want to see it, along with great body control. I will even go so far as to choose a song in my head and see myself dancing in perfect time to the beats of the music. In this visual program that I am creating, I can create mistakes, like a stumble, a forgotten step, or a memory that just goes blank, and view my reaction and corrections to the situation. I can imagine another dance couple bumping into us, and then picture myself regaining my composure and continuing on with the performance. I can view every detail and circumstance, as I wish it to be. Sometimes, in my head, I design a new dress that I would like to be wearing in the future. I like to picture myself as the winner at the end, smiling, and receiving the award.

I think that dancers like to see a mental rehearsal as they are in their body, and looking out toward the camera, or the audience. This is so helpful, as one is able to reinforce the feeling that goes along with each movement. Sometimes, we dancers are actually going over a dance routine in our head while in the midst of some other mundane activity. For instance, the long wait for luggage at the airport baggage claim often makes me want to take my mind somewhere else. As most travelers have their heads down, text messaging on their cell phones, I find myself drifting off into mental rehearsal of a dance routine, or some new step, or choreography that I am trying to memorize. Jim, will often catch me working on dance steps in the baggage claim area. He immediately recognizes what is going on and laughs as he inquires, "What are you working on?"

One time, I was deep in concentration, mentally rehearsing my Rumba routine, while staring blankly across the many baggage carousels at Washington DC's Dulles Airport. I naturally just began doing my Rumba steps, right there, in my Ugg boots no less. I was just kind of in a trance in my own head. When I finally snapped out of it, I caught eye contact with a man who had been watching me, and obviously thought I was nuts. Oh well, it was a wise use of time, and productive for me.

One day some ladies on my neighborhood tennis team were chatting about an odd woman who they had observed on daily walks with her Border Collie. They surmised that the woman must have Turrets Syndrome, as she sporadically kicked her leg out, and flung her arms up in the air. When I realized whom they were talking about, I could not contain my laughter.

"She does not have Turrets Syndrome," I informed them. "That's my friend, Debbie. She is a dancer. She is practicing her developés and rondés."

It was a long walk around that neighborhood, and an ideal time for Debbie to ponder her dance routines while throwing in a few steps here and there, and perfecting her technique.

Another dancer friend of mine, Michael, told me that he used to love to work on his dance technique while grocery shopping. One day he was practicing his Cuban hip action while doing Rumba walks and pushing his cart down aisle twelve, the frozen food section of the grocery store. Suddenly, a small boy, behind him shouted, "Mommy, that man is strange!" Michael had been completely caught up in his own world, oblivious to his surroundings.

The grocery store is such a great place for a dancer to practice Latin walks, because it offers a nice, smooth floor, long aisle ways, and the shopping cart! The shopping cart is like training wheels for a dancer. You can hang onto the cart for balance, and unlike a partner, the cart will not shout at you and say, "Stop hanging on me!"

The study of sports psychology can be so beneficial to dancers who recognize the importance of gaining mental fortitude. Ballroom dancing requires energy and strength, yet at the same time, the couples must show a picture of graceful movement that is tension-free, along with an air of confidence. The most skilled performance can be hindered by lack of mental strength and confidence. The study of sports psychology, along with the application of its techniques and tools, will improve and elevate the level of any dancer's performance.

>> **DARLA'S TIPS FOR**

## Overcoming Failure and Improving Your Performances

1. Do not put a time limit on your quest to win. "Often the struggler has given up, when he might have captured the victor's cup."

2. Remember that failure is not forever. Disappointments and setbacks make the satisfaction and joys of coming back and winning so much bigger and better.

3. Mental attitude has a direct impact on competitive performance. By learning to diagnose and monitor your own thoughts, you will be able to block out negative images, doubts, and fears.

4. Paint a mental picture of your winning performance.

5. Believe in yourself and your ensuing victory.

## Chapter 19

# The Spiritual Influence

You don't get what you hope for.
You don't get what you wish for.
You get what you believe.

**—Oprah Winfrey**

L ike many, I believe that a spiritual connection can enhance and maximize human potential. After reading the book, *The Secret*, several years ago, I became fascinated with this "law of attraction," that many of the greatest masters of the world regard as the most powerful law of the universe. The basic premise is that your current thoughts are creating your future life. When you focus on something, it happens to you because you are attracting it and calling it to existence. By learning to become the master of your own thoughts, you can control them and change them, thus change your life.

I remember feeling afraid and depressed for a few weeks after my hip replacement surgery. I still had pain and swelling, which made me feel fatigued and lazy. Unable to drive my car, I felt like a prisoner in my own home. I was having a hard time visualizing a positive, happy future.

In the past, when I was feeling down or lost, I reached for my DVD of *The Secret*. Having watched this video numerous times over the past few years, I always found myself feeling comforted and uplifted after seeing the masters and hearing their soothing voices relay their insights and stories.

One of my favorite parts is where John Assaraf talks about implementing the law of attraction by creating a "vision board." The idea is to put pictures of things that you want to achieve or attract on a board to be placed where you can see it every day. As you look at the images, daily, you concentrate and visualize yourself as having achieved or acquired these things. The law of attraction says that your thoughts become things. Most important is that you show gratitude for what you already have, and expect the things that you want to have in the future. John Assaraf described a vision board that he made on which he placed the photo of his dream house. Five years later, he was unpacking some forgotten old boxes and found the vision board. He had not realized until then that he had actually bought, renovated, and moved into the very house that he placed on his vision board.

I realized that I needed a vision board more than anyone. I knew that I could make myself feel better if I could visualize my recovery and my future achievements. My vision board would set and show my goals of what I wanted and expected to achieve with regards to my recovery and my dancing. I became so excited as I got ideas and put photos together for my vision board. There was so much work to do, and there would be no time left for any depression.

Assembling my vision board was such fun. My creativity really had me laughing at times. I started by putting up photos of my walker and my cane with big red exes through them to show that soon they would no longer be needed. I added photos of my favorite elliptical machine, and gym equipment, and then imposed photos of myself onboard. I got a photo of a woman body builder, and replaced her head with my own headshot. This was to show how strong I would become in the following months. My hip was still swollen, so I added a photo of myself in my tightest, skinniest jeans, which I was sure to be wearing in the future.

Jim and I like to spend a couple of days in Vegas every few months. The last time that we had been there, I had struggled to walk a couple of blocks down the street, and endured pain merely trying to make my way through a hotel lobby. After watching a stage show, I could barely manage to pull myself up and out of my chair to get up the steps to exit the theater. As I recalled the nagging joint pain that had ruined my fun, I put up a photo of the Vegas strip on my vision board. I added a photo of a jogger right in front of the Vegas photo. Of course, I cut off her head and replaced it with mine. A vision board requires a fair amount of decapitation of photos to create the perfect visual. Ha! I wanted to visualize myself running pain-free down the Vegas strip.

Most importantly, I added a few dancing photos of Jim and me. Underneath I wrote in big red letters: "Darla Davies—United States Pro Am American Smooth Champion. The first athlete in history to win a U.S. Championship with a hip replacement in a sport where you have to move your butt swiftly."

Every morning, after I woke up, I admired my vision board as I smiled and gave thanks. I chose to thank God for my new hip, along with my future recovery and victories to come. I do not think it matters much who you thank. If you do not believe in God, you can just give thanks to the universe, or whomever you choose to worship—Buddha, Allah, or the man in the moon. I think the important concept is just to be grateful for what you have and expect to receive good things, which will be drawn to you by your own thoughts.

My first year of dancing with my new hip went very well. Overall, I was pleased with my placements at the competitions and I had some good wins. At the U.S. Championships, I placed fifth. I cannot say that I was surprised or disappointed, because out of thirty entries, placing fifth in the nation is really quite good. I felt that I danced my personal best, so I was content and grateful that I, with my new hip, made it to the final round of seven couples.

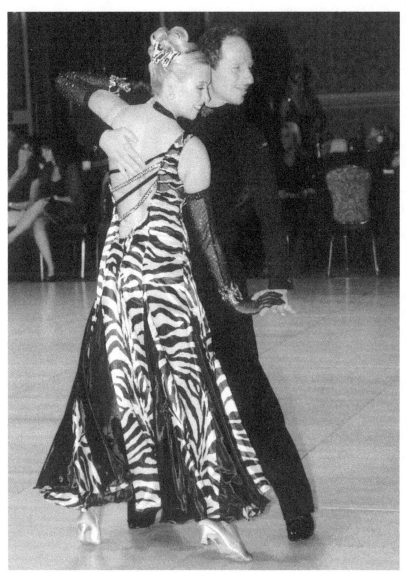

Living the dream. The first step to winning is believing that you can win.

Not too long after that I was watching my favorite pastor, Joel Osteen, deliver his weekly television sermon. That Sunday, Joel was encouraging us to give thanks to God, ask Him for what we want, be ready to receive it, and expect it. Joel suggested that if you really want something badly, you must live and act as though you *already* have it. Joel went on to explain that if you have negative thoughts or visions, your life will follow that direction. Your life will not change until you change the picture and view it as you want it to be.

"That's the secret!" I shouted at the television. "Joel is telling me to practice the secret!"

Perhaps I had not fully committed myself to believing and receiving during the past year. From that day on, I decided to follow Joel's advice with gusto. I began to live and believe in my dream, as if I had *already* won the championship. I told myself that I only needed to go dance in the event and pick up my trophy in September, because I was staking a claim on it right then and there, at that very moment. Unknowingly, Joel Osteen had just given me the best sports psychology tip ever! Some would call it arrogance, but I recall Dr. Rotella saying that arrogance can improve a performance and make you believe you can win. I had to do this. I had to eat, sleep, breathe, and believe every moment that I was already the 2011 Champion. I did a very good job of talking the talk.

I told Jim we should save that special, expensive bottle of champagne for after I win in September. I went to see Julia, my dressmaker, and for the first time tried on the dress that I would be wearing for the U.S. Championships in September. I felt as though I had just stepped into Dorothy's ruby slippers.

I smiled at Julia and said, "This dress is awesome! I know I will be a champion the first time that I dance in this dress."

During a workout with my personal trainer, Derek, I told him, "I really despise these exercises that you are making me do, but it's worth the pain and agony because this is what will help make me a champion in September."

A week before the U.S. Championships, at a competition in Los Angeles, I prepared the photographers for my big win as well. I told them, "Next week, I will be here at your booth looking at myself standing in front of the line, in my championship photo."

Everyone was so supportive and seemed to delight in skipping down the yellow brick road of my dream, right alongside me. They all knew that my planning was not arrogance. I had worked so hard to get back from hip replacement to fighting form. Everyone knew that this was my dream, and I was planning it and dreaming it my way.

Life is like a reality show and we are the players, so we must choose how we want things to transpire. I was so excited that I started preaching to anyone who would listen. I told friends that we must choose a positive picture and have faith in ourselves. When your vision is negative, your life will follow that direction. Your life will not change until you change the picture.

As Glenda the good witch told Dorothy, "You are wearing the ruby slippers. You have the power."

Oh, my goodness, even *The Wizard of Oz* was making perfect sense! You can turn your dreams into reality.

That line from the movie *Flashdance* has flashed through my mind so many times. *When you give up your dream, you die.* Of course there will always be ups and downs, and things are not always going to go your way. You must be committed to winning the battle within yourself, and keep yourself from giving in or giving up. I believe the hardest thing to do is to persevere to the top, because it is so much easier to just to settle for mediocrity or give up altogether.

This spiritual influence over my mental preparation for becoming a champion was like the icing on the sports psychology cupcake. It was a discovery that added joy and enhancement to my overall thinking regarding competition.

## DARLA'S TIP FOR

### Controlling Negative Thoughts

Negative thoughts will destroy your plan and attract the wrong things to you, so it is important to eliminate them immediately. You can chase bad thoughts away by trying to concentrate on things that make you feel good and happy. The second I feel a sad or defeating thought enter my head, I try to almost scare it away with my favorite biblical phrase: *No weapon formed against me shall prosper*. After saying this to myself, I feel powerful. I feel like I have just slayed the enemy.

## Chapter 20

# What Makes a Winner?

*Winners do things that losers don't want to do.*
**—Dr. Phil**

There are so many influences and factors that contribute to a winning ballroom dance performance. Surprisingly, the winner is often not the best dancer in the group, but the one who won the judges over with performance, personality, and overall look. Issues that go far beyond skill and technique often determine the winner.

In the big championship events, the judges are looking at the professional and amateur (Pro Am) team as a couple, however, heavy emphasis in their scoring is based on the performance of the amateur who is the student.

First impressions are so important in a ballroom dance performance. The judges are observing the contestants as they walk out onto the dance floor to take their beginning positions. Obviously, elegant walking with a confident smile, trumps clunky walking and a nervous expression or demeanor.

A dancer's appearance can turn off a judge. A dull or ill-fitting dress, along with any type of wardrobe malfunction including a hairdo that is unraveling, can leave a bad impression with the judges. A dancer's shoe flying off in the middle of a dance is also a negative distraction.

Certain elements of the dancing itself can also be a turn off to the educated eyes of the judges. Probably the most serious faux pas is a couple out of sync with each other and the music regarding timing and movement. Leading and following of movements should appear effortless.

Also unappealing is a couple that seems to fumble or forget their steps. Simply executing the choreography perfectly is not enough to assure a win at high-level competition. Dancing with feel and partner interaction is more impressive to a judge than just mechanically rehearsing a routine.

Ballroom dancers come from various backgrounds and often have participated in other types of dance or sports. Previous experiences often influence a dancer's ballroom dancing style. Ballroom dancers who have had a ballet background can spin like a top, do the splits, and bend over backwards, kicking a leg up to the sky. Moves like this combined with a big smile can be a favorable influence on some judges. Traditional, old school judges will contend that ballroom dancing is not *Cirque de Soleil,* and they will not be impressed by a dance routine full of such "tricks." Educated ballroom masters are more impressed by correct technique such as dividing and swinging of the legs while showing comfortable ease of movement from one leg to the other. This display of proper technique, combined with maintenance of balance and timing with the music, are the elements possessed by champion dancers. Also important is correct body alignment—a wide, uplifted dance frame that is free of tension—along with blunder-free dance steps.

Unfortunately, sometimes the winner of an event is the least technically proficient of the six finalists. Sometimes, a lady dancer will show a great upper body with animated arm styling, and a face that projects such joy that she is able to just draw the judges into her jubilant aura. Sadly, these enamored judges end up giving her a high mark, having never looked down at her feet, which are missing the basic technical heel leads, and flopping across the floor.

In essence, the winner of a ballroom dance championship event does not have to be the fastest spinner or a prima ballerina. A champion ballroom dancer can make up for what is lacking by putting forth extra effort into technique, musical timing, and strong movement, along with showing the character of each dance, and having a beautiful, overall presentation. A winner presents a package of many elements, not merely one or two.

Winning dancers do not walk away from a few weekly dance lessons thinking that is all it takes to make them a winner. Most students are not able to grasp new technique, styling, or choreography during a short lesson or two. It is necessary for the student to study and understand the material, and be able to physically produce the movements required, while maintaining mental control over the performance. Some dance students do nothing outside of their weekly lessons. Others go the extra mile by practicing their dance routines solo, engaging in fitness training, and studying sports psychology. There are those students who think that after a few lessons, all they have to do is put on a pretty dress, get their hair and makeup done, and they will become a winner. These individuals even go so far as to put a time limit on their quest to become a winner. They are the contestants who always cry and complain about their final placement, not able to comprehend why they did not end up five places higher. There is a simple explanation for this outcome: Winners do things that losers do not want to do. Becoming a winner takes time, effort, and work.

A great costume can certainly enhance a dancer's performance. I am a firm believer that a great dress can actually move a dancer up a place or two in the final lineup. There are some dresses that are undoubtedly what I call "first place" dresses. Color, design, fit, and movement on the

dance floor are the combined elements that make a dress spectacular—
or not. Sometimes I see a dress hanging on the sale rack, or even on the
body of a woman who is trying it on, and I will say to myself, *it looks
like a fifth place dress* or *it looks like a third place dress; not a winning dress.*

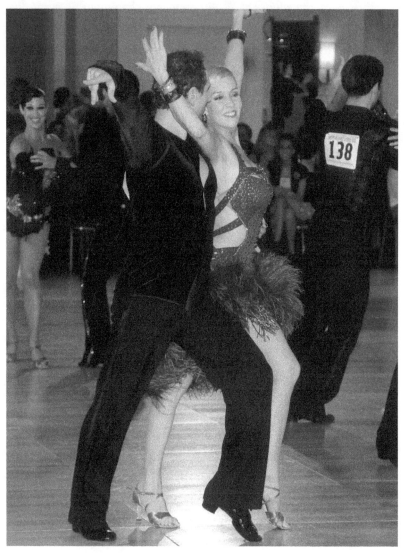

A spectacular costume shows great design, color, and movement.

When I see one of my feared competitors walk out onto the competition floor wearing a dress that looks obviously off in design or color, I heave a big sigh of relief. I call these dresses the "K.O.D. look"—that stands for kiss of death. Funny, but I am almost always right. The woman in the K.O.D. dress never wins. It does not require skill to spot one of these dresses. Sometimes they are a putrid shade of green or yellow, but oddly enough, I have seen some very unattractive plain white dresses. There is nothing more beautiful than a white gown that is done right.

Sometimes, the colors used in a particular dress are just unrelated, and sometimes the design has just too much going on—too many ideas on the same canvas. Other times, the gown is too simple, and it ends up looking like nothing more than a negligee, more suited for the bedroom. Some dancers try to be too sexy when they just do not have the body to pull it off. Too many women try to show too much skin when the best decision is to cover it up. I have seen many women who look like stuffed sausages in their dresses. It seems as though every woman has an inert desire to look sexy and wear a backless gown, but honestly, no one wants to see rolls of back fat. It is like going to a nude beach and seeing a bunch of overweight, out of shape bodies. You just want to run up to them and say, "Please, put your clothes back on!"

On the flip side, it can feel so threatening to see a competitor walk out onto the dance floor wearing a knockout, gorgeous dress. A great dress helps a dancer standout among her competitors and draw in the focus of the judges. Many times, I have seen a professional female dancer competing in a dress that I found to be visually mesmerizing. It is a big advantage being able to see a dress dance, and move on the floor, before you buy it. These particular gowns are usually always for sale, because the pro dancers are sponsored by various dressmakers. I have purchased quite a few of my dresses literally right off of the back of a pro dancer.

With a few alterations, or none at all, the dress got a new owner, and I got a new look.

The one element a dancer cannot control in her efforts to put down a winning performance is the judging panel. All that a competitor can do is pray for a fair and unbiased panel of judges. Unfortunately, there are political influences in ballroom dancing competitions. Many of the judges are also organizers of competitions. Such a judge might give generous marks toward a friend or pro competitor, in hopes of enticing him or her to bring many competing students to that judge's competition later in the year. It is like the judge is saying, "I will scratch your back now, if you will come and scratch mine later." Judges also coach many of the professional and amateur competitors. Sadly, there is a perception that these judges may favor their own paying clients/students.

A ballroom dance judge is paid for his opinion, which can be based on practically anything. Any judge can come up with a preference, area of focus, or a reason for marking one couple over another. The most highly respected judges will show no political preferences. A judge of integrity will tell you that the marks on his or her judging card will not be influenced by the fact that you are best friends, or just had lunch together. If he or she is judging you in a dance competition, it is the dancing that will be assessed, and you will be given the placement that you deserve, even if it is last place.

Another factor to be considered is that not every judge on the panel sees every step of every routine being performed by each couple. For instance, in a six couple final round of an event, each couple may have seconds of brilliance in their routines, and then other points that are a bit dull or lacking. If more than a couple of judges miss the exciting parts of a couple's performance, and instead witness a blunder, then favor will likely be directed toward the other competitors.

Sometimes, when Jim and I are preparing to walk out onto the competition floor, I will ask him, "Is this judging panel good, bad, or ugly?"

We laugh about my silly question, but it is actually kind of sad. Often we can look at a judging panel and predict my placement in the event, before we ever walk out onto the floor and do the actual dancing. If I know that three or four of my competitors each have two or three coaches on the judging panel, it will not be a good day for me. Sad as this might be, I refuse to get hung up on the situation. My only goal is to go out onto the competition floor and dance my personal best. I want to show the judges why they should mark me first; I want them to feel guilty and like they have made a mistake if they choose not to mark me first.

The judging panel is always going to be a crapshoot. Competitors who feel they are out of the loop politically can opt to follow one of two paths.

- ☐ **Option one** is that they can run around the country and get coaching from as many judges as possible. Unless one owns a Learjet, this plan will probably empty one's bank account.
- ☐ **Option two**, and the one I stand by, is to just wow the judges with good, quality dancing. What a challenge and an accomplishment it is to entice judges to give you good marks when it was originally not part of their plans. They might want to ignore you, but if your dancing is good, they will be forced to look your way.

Over the past several years, there was one particular judge who used to always mark me dead last. After I started competing again with my new hip, I saw her familiar face on several judging panels.

This judge ran into Jim one day and said to him, "You know, I never used to mark Darla, but I do now. She has really improved. Her dancing is a lot better."

When Jim relayed their conversation to me, I was overjoyed. In years past, not only were my skills, timing, and balance not evolved, but my fluidity of dancing was marred by my deteriorating hip joint. I am sure that my dancing performance had been undeserving of that judge's mark. I never had the opportunity to receive coaching from this lady, so clearly there was no obligation for her to even look twice at me. However, after this judge saw me dance a couple of times with my new hip, she did start to see me in a different light. The improvement in the quality of my dancing and performance forced this judge to see me in a new light! That one comment, made casually in passing that one day, meant so much to me and made me believe that I could make it to the top.

Dancers come in all shapes and sizes, and some are obviously more talented than others, yet all possess some appealing quality that is special and unique to that individual. Some are more athletic, whereas others are more artistic. Some are lacking in technical mastery, yet they put out great emotion and energy in their dancing. Then there might be a dancer who is sort of like a jack-of-all-trades; someone who is not super fabulous at any one aspect, but pretty darn good at many elements. The spectrum of appealing qualities in a dancer is like a rainbow of many colors. I believe that there is something beautiful about every dancer, and each one should try to develop their best qualities.

Singers are often encouraged not to copy another singer's style, but to focus on developing more of an individual style. On the television show *American Idol*, the judges commend the singing contestants for "knowing who they are," or "being true to who they are." The judges like it when the contestants put their own spin on a famous song rather than mimic the superstar who originally recorded the song. The same principle applies in ballroom dancing. What works for one dancer's style might not look so good on another dancer. When a dancer tries to be like someone else, instead of herself, the consequences can be disastrous.

Several years ago, Jim had a student who had won a U.S. championship in the American Smooth division. She presented an elegant look with her classic red dress and her dark chocolate brown hair coiffed into a sleek updo. The following year, this lady placed third in the same event at the national championships. That was still a great result, and nothing to frown about, because as we all know, nobody wins all of the time.

Jim's student continued to let her frustration agitate her into the next year as a particular tall, lean blonde who had an ultrashort haircut was winning most of her events, week after week. Jim's student thought that if she made her own look resemble that of her dominating competitor, the judges would once again love her and make her a winner. The transformation began with chopping off her long dark hair. The once elegant updo was replaced with what I call a frumpy, short, "housewife hairdo." Needless to say this change only made this lady's look less appealing, not more appealing.

Prior to the national championships the following year, Jim's student dyed her frumpy, housewife hair blond. In her mind, that hair was going to make her a standout in the eyes of the judges. She traded in the elegant gowns for a bright yellow dress with fluttery sleeves that made her look like a frumpy canary. It did not matter how this lady danced because her look was so off that the essence of who she was as a dancer was lost.

After dropping to fifth at the nationals, this lady's attitude went from sour to rotten. The downward spiral continued as she eventually went on to blame her bad competition results on her teacher. Having moved on to a new teacher, the poor lost soul dyed her hair red and purchased some new competition gowns. The quality of her dancing dwindled, and she found herself unable to make it to the finals at competitions where she had won in previous years. This once elegant champion self-destructed, fizzled out, and quit altogether. Instead of trying to improve her skills while staying true to who she was as a dancer, this lady became consumed with adopting someone else's look, which ultimately led to her downfall.

## Darla's Advice to Dance Competitors

You have a quality that is special and unique to you as a person and as a competitor. Stay true to who you are rather than try to morph into some other character. There is nothing wrong with diversifying your own look, but adopting someone else's appearance will not make you more talented or more deserving. Concentrate on your own special strengths and abilities. Believe in yourself.

## Chapter 21

# Destiny at Disney

To triumph over hardship is the journey
of the American dream.

**—Laura Hillenbrand**

Competing at the U.S. DanceSport Championships makes many dancers tense. It is the ultimate challenge and an honor to win a U.S Championship title in the world of ballroom dancing. Amateur dancers, like me, are every bit as competitive as the professional dancers. Winning can mean so much to some that they do not even show up to dance at this competition for fear of losing. It is easier for one to say, "My schedule would not allow me to compete at the U.S. Championships," rather than have to say, "I danced at the U.S. Championships and lost." I always want to win as much as the rest of them, but I am not afraid of losing, because I accept that nobody is at the top all the time. One must have the guts to put oneself out there and plan for victory, yet be accepting of defeat. You cannot win the lottery if you do not buy a ticket.

The 2011 U.S. DanceSport Championships were held in Orlando, Florida, at Disney World's Swan Hotel. Having prepared for this day with high expectations, I was ready to throw them all away, relax, and enjoy the experience. How could one not feel joy in the land of Mickey and Minnie Mouse—the Magic Kingdom?

I wanted to be the first ballroom dancer (perhaps the first athlete of all time) with an artificial hip to win a U.S. Championship title in a sport requiring traveling movement. After months of preparation for this day, I was feeling confident, focused, and composed. I imagined that I was wearing Dorothy's ruby slippers, knowing inside myself that I had the power to win. I was ready to create my own reality.

Years ago as an equestrian competitor, I found the technique of mental rehearsal to be both comforting and beneficial. As a ballroom dancer, I find this technique to be extremely useful and relaxing as well. The day before my event, I visually rehearsed all of my dance routines in my head several times. I imagined Jim and myself walking out onto the floor for the final round of my big scholarship event. I pictured us dancing the Waltz, Tango, Foxtrot, and Viennese Waltz with perfect timing and technique. I thought about the challenging spots in each routine, and went over them reciting the timing, "one and two, three, one, two, three" or "quick, quick, quick, and slow." I pictured myself moving with speed and power across the dance floor, completely in sync with Jim, while maintaining a lifted, wide dance frame.

As I had done hundreds of times before, I was creating my own movie. I viewed the film in my head. I edited out mistakes, and even pictured myself coping with difficulties and problems. I imagined how I would react if another couple bumped into us in the middle of a dance. I pictured myself regaining my composure and timing, and continuing on with the dance, unflustered. Going over the dance routines in my head several times kept them fresh in my mind and helped me to remember some recent changes and additions to the choreography and technique.

I looked forward to the happy feelings that I would soon be experiencing with a magnificent win. I pictured Jim helping me up to the number one platform, and standing beside me, both of us smiling for the championship photo. I even pictured myself later that evening, celebrating, and drinking champagne with my friends.

Jim and I both felt it would be a good idea to run through our dance routines and feel the floor prior to the competition. Often a dance floor can be sticky in some spots, and slick in others. Sometimes the entire floor feels slippery. Events were scheduled to begin in the ballroom at seven o'clock that morning, and Jim had several other students to rehearse with as well. I went down to the ballroom for my rehearsal with Jim at five-thirty. After a few sips of self-brewed, hotel room coffee and some brief warm up stretches, we danced our Waltz. Music would have been nice and helpful, but unfortunately, it was not available for this practice session. I felt as though my waltz around the room was pretty good, however Jim's facial expression reflected a different assessment of the quality of my dancing. I do not remember ever having a stellar early morning practice before a competition, so Jim's disappointment in the situation was no surprise to me.

As I had heard numerous times in the past, Jim told me that I was "stumbling" and "not on my feet." In the past, these comments used to alarm and fluster me. Jim is tougher and more demanding on me than with his other students, because as a married couple, he knows he can use words to provoke me and make me try harder. He knew how badly I wanted to win this title, and he wanted it every bit as much for me.

In the past, when Jim would tell me that I was "not on my feet," I would reply, "Well, whose feet am I on?" I knew that this sarcasm would irritate him, so I opted out of that reply this time. Instead, I used the excuse that I had just been dragged out of bed at five AM, which was not conducive to great dancing. He was somewhat sympathetic, however, he did not return my smile. I assured Jim that I would be able to pull it all together for my events later that afternoon. I asked him to just be patient, help me work on a few things, and just finish the practice with a positive feeling. Jim and I completed all four of the American Smooth dances with several stops and starts. After a few reminders and corrections on position and technique, I finished the practice session feeling strong and ready to take on the competition.

I had a few hours to eat breakfast, get my hair and makeup done, and enjoy my double shot soy mocha. I did more stretching and limbering up exercises in the hotel room. While stretching my legs on the bureau, I performed the four dance routines in my head once again, as I stared blankly at the wall. Next, I walked through parts of each routine, right there in that small narrow strip of hotel room space, in my sweat pants and socks. I stood in front of the mirror above the desk, and made various dance frame poses.

Feeling good, I put on my silk, zebra-print ball gown, and proceeded down to the ballroom. Jim was competing with a couple of his other students, so I just sat down, relaxed, and watched for a few minutes. About fifteen minutes prior to my dance events, I got up and started to do some stretching and swinging of my legs.

These preliminary heats are often used by many of us as a warm up for the big scholarship championship at the end of the day. The results of these early events can be completely different, or opposite to those occurring later in the day under a different and larger judging panel. We might not like politics in judging of ballroom dancing, but unfortunately it is part of the sport. Judges are paid to give their opinions, whatever those opinions might be, and whatever the basis for those opinions. I always hope for a judging panel that will just look at the dancing and mark it as they see it on that day. Sadly, I have often looked at a judging panel before I walked out onto the floor, and accurately predicted my upcoming placement in that event. I wish I were not that smart.

I competed in two sets of single dance events, dancing the Waltz, Tango, Foxtrot, and Viennese Waltz. I was awarded one first, five seconds, and two thirds. A clean sweep would have been preferred, but I was not displeased or upset with those results. I still believed that I could, and would, be a U.S. Champion later that day. Nobody knew what judging panel would be up there for the final round of my big scholarship event. In my mind, I just chose to dream my dream and make plans for everything to go my way.

 **DARLA'S TIPS FOR**

## Competitors

1. Sometimes you will give a great performance, perhaps your best ever, and still not be the winner. Remember, if you have given your best, you are a winner regardless of the outcome.

2. Keep your focus on being the best that you can be, rather than trying to beat others.

## Chapter 22

# One Moment in Time

Give me one moment in time
When I'm more than I thought I could be
When all of my dreams are a heartbeat away
And the answers are all up to me
Give me one moment in time
When I'm racing with destiny
Then in that one moment in time
I will feel
I will feel eternity

**—Albert Hammond and John Bettis**

A couple of hours later I was back in the hotel room, this time slipping into my new tiger-print ball gown. As a lover of animal prints, I had been competing throughout the year in both my leopard-print and my zebra-print gowns. Both dresses looked magnificent out on the dance floor and under the lights. Each one brought so many compliments.

A few months prior to the Orlando competition, I told my dressmaker, Julia, about my great idea for a new dress. "I already have leopard and zebra, so what do you think about tiger for the U.S. Championships?" I inquired.

Julia agreed that the tiger choice would be fantastic. We held a swatch of the tiger fabric alongside various colored fabrics, searching for the best accent color to use on the dress. We easily agreed that the bright turquoise silk looked stunning against the copper shade of the Lycra® tiger print. After a brief discussion regarding the details of the design, I could not wait to see the finished product.

There I stood in front of the hotel room mirror, admiring Julia's finished masterpiece. The tiger and turquoise fabric sparkled under hundreds of Swarovski crystals. Swarovski stoned copper and turquoise rings circled my neck and across my bare back. The matching stoned circle bracelets on top of my long, sheer turquoise gloves added the perfect accent to the dress. My hair stylist had woven a turquoise piece of synthetic hair throughout my blond updo. It was such a fun and unique final touch to go with my matching bronze and turquoise eye shadow. The entire picture was breathtaking to me.

As I entered the ballroom, this spectacular dress and hairdo made me feel as though I could take on anything. My sports psych mind was prepared and focused, having let go of my memories of my second and third place finishes earlier that afternoon. The top contenders were present, so I knew that it was not going to be an easy battle. I had to keep my mind on track with my plan.

I proceeded over to the table where Jim's students were relaxing in between their heats during the competition. A lady complimented me on my dress as I made my way around the room, past some other tables. Knowing I had about an hour or so before we would be dancing, I just stood at the back of the ballroom and did some light stretching and moving around. I did not want to just sit in a chair and get too

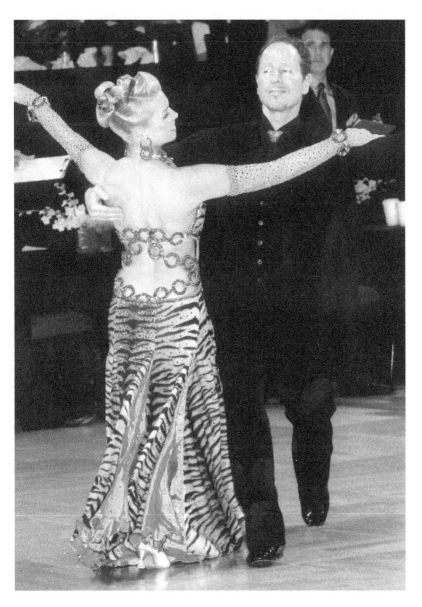

My spectacular dress and hairdo made me feel like a winner.

relaxed. I wanted to be limber and sharp. I was not feeling nervous, but I was really ready to get on with the task. If racehorses can think, they probably have similar feelings of anticipation as they walk onto the track and move toward the starting gate for a race.

I flexed my knees and sunk my body weight into my legs. At the same time, I raised and lifted my upper body and practiced contracting and releasing my back muscles. I took a series of steps side-to-side, and then forward and back. I was concentrating on sinking my center of gravity into the floor from the waist down as I levitated my upper body from the waist up. I wanted to feel a strong, solid, connection with the floor as I moved.

*Uh Oh. Crap!* I stepped on the bottom of my dress a couple of times as I was moving around. *Not good. What if it is too long?* I thought. I had had a couple of fittings with this dress, but had not done much more than take a few steps and twirl around several times in front of a mirror. In fact, I had not even seen the finished product until the dress was brought to me the previous day. I remembered a couple of times in the past, when I had stepped on the hems of dresses during competitions. Once, I was doing the Viennese Waltz at the prestigious Ohio Star Ball competition and stepped on the silk skirt of my dress. I was on the ground before I even knew what had happened. Jim pulled me up, and we just continued on with the dance like nothing had ever happened. The whole incident passed so quickly that it was likely missed by most of the judges.

I certainly did not want that to happen again. *Not now. Not here! Ugh, I cannot obsess over this; I have to deal with it. I must take control over this situation. I will not allow myself to step on this dress and fall. It is just simply not an acceptable option.*

Julia and I had discussed the technique of "working the skirt" on the zebra dress that I had been wearing for the last four months. While dancing, the lady reaches down and takes hold of her skirt somewhere above the knee. She proceeds to dance, with skirt in hand for a few bars of music. If done smoothly and gracefully, the artistry of movement

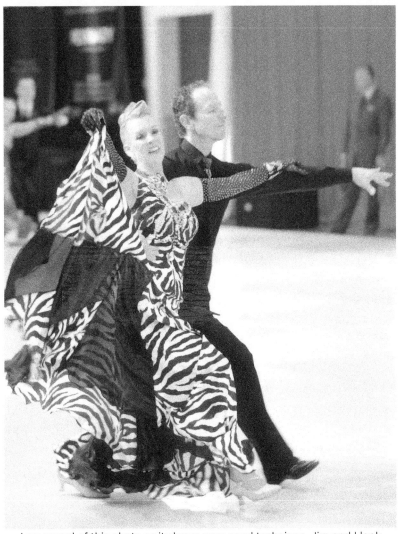

I am proud of this photo as it shows very good technique. Jim and I look
in sync as our heels are simultaneously striking the floor, and my skirt
looks beautiful in my hand.

combined with a gorgeous patterned skirt can be visually captivating.
This simple display seems to be a lost art nowadays. I have not noticed
many amateur dancers even making an attempt to work it into their

routines. I had been practicing with my other dress for a few months, and I had done a pretty good job. The skirt on the new tiger gown had a lot more material. The voluminous Lycra® skirt with silk insets was much heavier than the light silk skirt on my zebra gown. With slippery gloves on, it was going to be much more difficult to reach down and grab a hold of this skirt. I knew that it would be important to get a decent chunk of the skirt and grab it in the right place to hoist it up. In addition, I had to remember the parts in my routines where I wanted to "dance the skirt," so that I could be thinking about it, and prepare in advance to start reaching down. *Yikes, I already have enough on my mind.*

I started running through my dance routines in my head again, making mental note of all the places where I wanted to work my skirt. *There is that place in the Waltz, where I do the standing spin. Yes, it looks so good on that step. There is that diagonal line in the Tango, where it would look so good. I will try to remember to grab the skirt before we take off running. The Foxtrot is fine, but the Viennese Waltz is going to be crucial. I need to grab that skirt immediately after the intro. It's the last dance, and this first section of my routine will be so stunning with skirt in hand. I can't mess this up. I can't slip and fall. I won't slip and fall.*

I knew that there was about to be a change of the judging panel, because I noticed that the current one had been out there for nearly two hours. As my eyes followed the line of nine judges, I was thankful that a change was coming up soon. I silently prayed, *God, please just let us get a fair, impartial, non-political judging panel, and let me dance to the best of my ability. That's all I ask for…I accept whatever the results are going to be…whatever is meant to be…*

I knew that the stars would have to pretty much line up just right for me to win this thing. I knew they could just as well line up for one of the five other contestants in the final six, instead of me. That is assuming I would make it to the final round. I chose not to dwell on any negative thoughts and I proceeded on with my plan of being the winner.

A fresh, finely dressed, panel of judges made their way out onto the dance floor. I was pleasantly surprised. As far as I knew, none of these judges coached any of the top dancers in my group. Some of the judges were strangers to me, which I considered a positive. If they had not judged much throughout the year, maybe they did not know who the top couples were, which meant they would have no preconceived opinions or obligations, and just judge the dancing as they saw it that day. Getting over-analytical, I saw two judges who knew me, and also knew of my hip replacement. *What if they are going to assume I could not be as good with a new hip? Stop*! I had to stop analyzing the judges, forget it all, and just dance!

There were twenty-five competitors in our American Smooth Scholarship, so everyone knew that there would be three rounds of dancing. Those of us who would be lucky enough to make it to the final round would be dancing the Waltz, Tango, Foxtrot, and Viennese Waltz, three times.

As we walked out to the dance floor for the first round of the prestigious U.S. Championship, I felt remarkably relaxed. *Just listen to the music,* I thought. I gave myself an assignment to just ignore the other competitors and show the judges my personal best dancing. Jim—referred to as Mr. Smooth, the master of Pro Am competition—was not the one to worry about in this partnership. Although the judges observe and mark the overall performance of the couple in Pro Am dancing, most of the focus including the placement is rendered to the amateur who is the student. Judges will not favor an amateur student showing improper or poor technique, or lack of energy or movement. I needed to demonstrate that I could hold it all together. I had to show those judges that I was confident, competent, happy, and relaxed. Any inkling of tension or stress would not be a good thing.

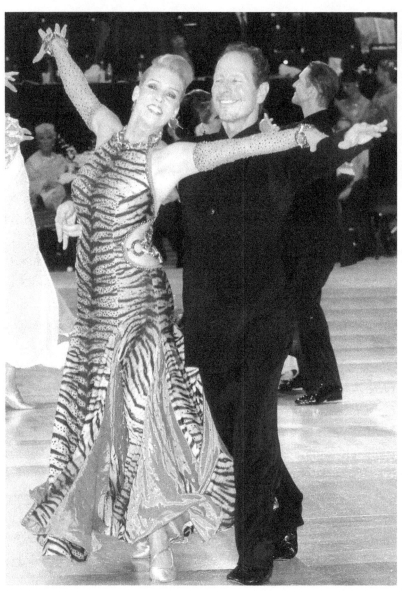

Through each round of dancing, I just felt happy to be dancing at the U.S. Championships, as I maintained my wide, uplifted dance frame.

The first round was going well until I had a wardrobe malfunction during my second dance—the Tango. My left glove had slipped down from my upper arm to below my elbow. *Damn!* I was irritated and shocked, because I had applied so much of that sticky body glue to my biceps before pulling the gloves on. *How could this happen?* I was just thankful that it happened on the first round and not during the final round! The judges would certainly not forgive a distraction like that in the final. It was distracting to me as well, but I had to ignore it, and just focus on my next two dances. Wardrobe malfunction aside, the first round went well. As soon as we exited the dance floor, I made a beeline over to our table to retrieve my body glue. As I liberally applied the slimy, sticky glue all up and down my arms, I thought, *there is no way I am going to let these things fall down again. I am here to win a U.S. Championship. Champions do not have wardrobe malfunctions!*

A few minutes later we were in the on-deck area waiting to hear the call back numbers for the semi-final round. I felt confident that we would make it into the next round, so I was feeling calm and collected.

As we began our semi-final round Waltz, I thought, *relax and stay with the music, keep your arms in a wide frame, and hold yourself up.* With only twelve couples on the floor this time, I wanted to show the judges that I was an obvious choice to mark through to the final round. After completing our four dances once again, I remained confident and relaxed as we exited the floor.

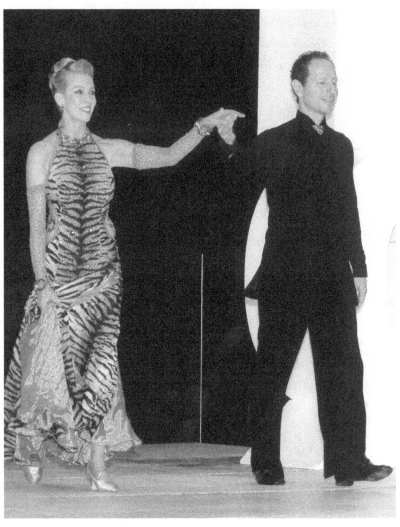

Walking down from the stage for our final round of dancing, I picked up my skirt to avoid tripping while my mind kicked into power mode.

We had a few minutes, once again, to cool off and get a drink of water before regrouping in the on-deck area to find out which six couples had made it to the final round. Yolanda, the deck captain, approached

Jim and motioned for us to line up back stage. Although we expected to make it to the final, it was still a relief when the word was given.

As the six couples assembled back stage, I noticed that the lady who had placed above me in all but one of the heats earlier that day was missing! I pointed out my observation to Jim. That was the lady who I had felt was the biggest threat to me in this competition, because she had placed above me numerous times over the past few years. There were still three ladies in this group, who had recently placed above me at past competitions. There was even a lady from Moscow who had beaten me quite handily two months prior at the Manhattan competition. That was the one and only time that we had ever danced against each other. *And there's a Russian judge on the panel. Crap!*

At this point, we were about two minutes away from walking onto the stage, down the steps, and onto the floor under the spotlights. My mind kicked into power mode. *I'm wearing the ruby slippers. I have the power. Everyone else is dancing for second place.* Next, my counseling from pastor Joel Osteen kicked in to gear. *No weapon formed against me shall prosper. Thank you God for making me a champion. I am here to receive your favor and my victory today.*

The next five or six minutes of dancing would seal our fate. One of the six of these couples would soon be standing on the top platform as the new champions—I so wanted it to be Jim and me.

As the couples spread out across the expansive dance floor and we took our positions for the first dance, I caught a glimpse of Miss Moscow out of the corner of my eye. I felt the butterflies. *No problem. Butterflies are good*, I thought. I remembered Dr. Rotella telling us that butterflies are the adrenalin that gives one strength and concentration. The greatest concern for a veteran athlete is when the butterflies are not there anymore. I wondered if Sea Biscuit had felt butterflies when he walked onto the racetrack and saw War Admiral prancing around before their historic match race. Certainly Roger Federer must feel butterflies when he sees Raphael Nadal come onto the tennis court and take his place on the other side of the net.

Letting go of all of the mental issues, I put my focus on looking energetic, happy, and relaxed once again. Some dancers get fatigued after dancing in many events throughout a day of competition, and one can easily lose their mojo by the time they get to the third round of their last event.

I thought our final Waltz was perhaps a personal best for me. It is difficult to feel the music and stay on time while remaining in sync with one's partner. If I get through a Waltz without Jim whispering to me, "listen to the music," then I know it was a good one. I had my dress in hand on the standing spin and I know it had to look great. Our Tango and Foxtrot were solid, and showed both good technique and character of the dances. We wrapped it up with our Viennese Waltz, and my legs felt so good and strong as I was traveling down the dance floor, transferring my weight from one leg to the other. I was able to get my skirt in hand at all of the right places. It almost felt as though we were flying towards home base or running toward the finish line of a very long race. I was floating with glee.

As we walked off the dance floor, I was excited because I felt that I had danced my best round ever, and I was content. At that point I knew that everything else was out of my control. Our fate was going to be determined by the opinions of those nine judges. Whether we dancers agreed or disagreed, we would have to accept the results. There would be no disputes, such as in tennis when a player can dispute a bad line call, or a jockey can dispute a result by claiming an intentional foul from another rider.

Jim danced a couple of more heats with his other students and I went back at our table again, where I chilled out for a few minutes. Having anticipated this dancing performance for so many months, I was very happy with the experience, yet also relieved that it was over.

As an advanced dancer who is partnered with a top professional, I felt the pressure to show excellence. Although many people had no knowledge of my hip replacement and struggle back to this top level of competition, they also had no knowledge of my lofty goal of winning this U.S. Championship. I had put a lot of stress on myself by living and believing in this dream for the past many months. The pressure gave me incentive to keep pressing onward with the strength training, the coaching, and pursuit of the title. This prize would make up for the memories of agony and pain.

Finally, the announcer started calling the dancers back up to the dance floor for the awards ceremonies. Jim's intermediate student placed second in her championship, and his senior student placed sixth in her event. As she was expressing her discontentment with her placement to Jim, the announcer called the competitors of my event to the dance floor for the awards.

*Ugh.* My stomach felt sick. I did not want to end up in fifth or sixth place. I did not even want to be second, third, or fourth. We all lined up across the dance floor, facing the announcer, and the podium where two of the judges were waiting to hand out the medals and the prize checks. The announcer began to call out the placements in reverse order.

"In sixth place, from Moscow…"

*What?* I was shocked, yet thrilled. I really expected to see that lady more toward the front of the line. Wow, the two most threatening ladies were already gone! I gave a small nervous sigh of relief.

"In fifth place, from California…"

Yes, one California dancer was gone. But there was an even better dancing lady from California standing right next to me. Dorothy must have felt this uneasiness when she thought the wicked old witch was dead, only to find that her sister, the wicked witch of the west was still alive. "And she's worse than the other one" were Glenda's daunting words, which also applied to this situation. In the case of the two Miss

California's in this event, the one remaining was a worse threat to me than the one who had just left the floor. *Oh hurry up,* I thought, *but don't call our number next.*

"In fourth place, from California…"

*Are you kidding me?* I had to force myself to keep breathing. I was both surprised and relieved that that one was gone, however, I was deeply concerned about the remaining Miss Minnesota standing on my left. I did not know much about the lady from Tennessee standing to my right. I had watched her dance in some heats earlier in the day. She was very attractive, and a beautiful dancer.

"In third place, from Tennessee…"

My heart was pounding. They were all gone except for Miss Minnesota and me. Three weeks prior, in the Las Vegas competition, this lady was the big winner. I had placed a disappointing fourth. Within the next twenty seconds, I was going to be either jubilant or dejected. I was about to hear one of two things: Either, "From M-m-m-m" for Minnesota, or "From A-a-a-a" for Arizona. *Please, Please, let him say Minnesota,* I willed. I was clenching tightly onto Jim's arm. The announcer continued. "And ladies and gentlemen, the runner up…" A long, lingering pause followed. I held my breath.

"From M-m-m-m-inesota…"

*He said it! He said Minnesota! Did I really hear Minnesota?* I looked at Jim.

"Did I really just win?" I asked.

"You did," he answered with a smile.

I was overcome with the exploding joy of that moment in time. Simultaneously smiling and crying, I hugged and kissed Jim. I jumped up and down in front of him about twenty times in a semi-circle, from his left side to his right side.

"Ladies, and gentlemen, your winners, from Phoenix, Arizona, Darla Davies with Jim Maranto!"

We walked forward and bowed to the audience as they applauded. I was crying as the Russian judge placed the medal around my neck. How I wished that my Mom and Dad could have been there to enjoy this victory with me. I knew they were watching from Heaven, but I really wanted to see the excitement and the joy on their faces.

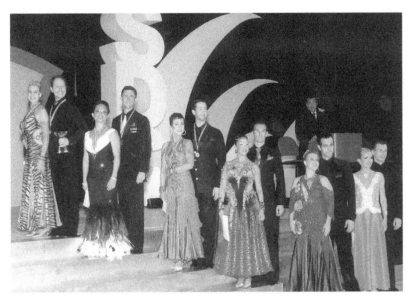

My one moment in time.

One of the photographers, sharing in my happiness, cutely asked if I could stop crying for his photo. After that, we were ushered to the top step on the stage for the official photo. There I was, living my dream. I was the 2011 Pro Am American Smooth Champion. My destiny. My one moment in time.

# Afterword

Each year since the writing of this book, Darla and Jim have continued to compete and win numerous ballroom dance championships throughout the country. Darla and Jim have consistently placed in the top six of her division at the United States Championships when able to compete. Jim is often asked to be a member of the highly respected judging panel, an honor that excludes him from participating as a competitor.

In 2014, Darla was once again sidelined from the dance floor with thyroid cancer. Before the surgery, Darla requested of her surgeon, "Please make this your best work, because I am scheduled to dance at a competition in Baltimore sixteen days from right now!"

The surgeon, laughed and said, "I will do my best to get you there."

In spite of what numerous nurses thought was possible, Darla and Jim did make it to that Baltimore competition. Although, not feeling one hundred percent, Darla was able to win two big events at that competition.

Darla always says, "I just try to get over the hurdles and keep going. Presently, Darla is still training hard at the gym and on the dance floor, believing that she can win more United States Championships in the future. Darla loves her titanium hip and says, "The more I beat this thing up the stronger and better it gets!"

# About the Author

At age forty, Darla felt burned out on the equestrian scene she been a part of for twenty-five years. After watching a ballroom dancing competition on television, Darla became enamored with the sport. Swing dance lessons at a community center led Darla to a small local ballroom studio and a dance camp where she met her future husband, Jim Maranto; a two-time professional American Smooth Ballroom Dance Champion.

Over the next several years, Darla won many awards as she progressed from beginner to the advanced level of ballroom dance competitions. In 2006, Darla and Jim performed on *America's Ballroom Challenge*, which was co-hosted by Marilu Henner and televised on PBS.

Years of sporting activities had robbed Darla of cartilage in her left hip. In 2008, Darla and Jim felt lucky to win the coveted U.S. Pro Am American Smooth Championship, in spite of Darla's weak left leg. No longer able to endure the joint pain that continued after numerous failed therapies and treatments, Darla succumbed to hip replacement surgery in 2009.

After being told by one surgeon that she would not be able to dance "like that again" after hip surgery, Darla kept searching until she found Dr. Anthony Hedley who gave Darla a new titanium hip, along with the confidence and courage to follow her dream of winning another national ballroom dance championship.

Darla fought her way back through the doubts and fears, as well as the physical challenges of rehabilitation and strength training. One year and ten months after hip replacement surgery, Darla partnered with husband Jim Maranto, became the 2011, U.S. Pro Am Smooth Champion.

As of this writing, she still continues to win at one championship after another.

## Follow Darla on Instagram at

https://www.instagram.com/AuthorDarlaDavies/

## Find Darla on Facebook at

https://www.facebook.com/AuthorDarlaDavies

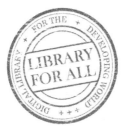